Current Issues in Toxicology

Current Issues in Toxicology

Sponsored by the
International Life Sciences Institute

Edited by H.C. Grice

Interpretation and Extrapolation of Chemical and
Biological Carcinogenicity Data to Establish
Human Safety Standards

The Use of Short-Term Tests for Mutagenicity and
Carcinogenicity in Chemical Hazard Evaluation

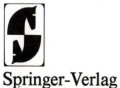

Springer-Verlag
New York Berlin Heidelberg Tokyo

H.C. Grice, *Editor*
Nepean, Ontario, Canada

© 1984 by Springer-Verlag New York Inc.

Media conversion by Ampersand, Rutland, Vermont.
Printed and bound by R.R. Donnelley & Sons, Harrisonburg, Virginia.
Printed in the United States of America.

9 8 7 6 5 4 3 2 1

ISBN 0-387-13696-7   Springer-Verlag   New York Berlin Heidelberg Tokyo
ISBN 0-540-13696-7   Springer-Verlag   Berlin Heidelberg New York Tokyo

Foreword

The International Life Sciences Institute (ILSI) is a scientific foundation which addresses critical health and safety issues of national and international concern. ILSI promotes international cooperation by providing the mechanism for scientists from government, industry and universities to work together on cooperative programs to generate and disseminate scientific data. The members and trustees of the Institute believe that questions regarding health and safety are best resolved when scientists can examine and discuss issues, as an independent body, separate from the political pressures of individual countries and the economic concerns of individual companies.

Frequently, meaningful assessment of the risk of a test substance is hindered by the inherent inconsistencies in the system. The development and refinement of methods and systems to evaluate the safety of chemicals have evolved in a rapid and largely unplanned fashion.

Attempts to improve the system have largely been directed toward broad general concerns, with little attention being given to specific problems or issues. A failure to resolve these problems has frequently resulted in increased testing costs and complications in the assessment and extrapolation of the results. Publicity surrounding toxicologic issues has created chronic public apprehension about the ability of science and government to deal effectively with these problems.

In response to these difficulties, ILSI has assembled highly qualified and renowned scientists from research institutes, universities, government and industry, with relevant scientific knowledge and expertise regarding the issues that complicate risk assessment procedures.

This series, *Current Issues in Toxicology*, is the result of the endeavors of these international scientists in this regard. It also exemplifies the commitment of ILSI to promote a better understanding of critical safety issues. Throughout this series, an attempt is made to not only examine the factors which influence the evaluation of the safety of chemicals but also to develop principles, recommend guidelines and define areas requiring additional research.

Contents

Current Issues in Toxicology

Interpretation and Extrapolation of Chemical and Biological Carcinogenicity Data to Establish Human Safety Standards

Editor in Chief
Dr. Harold C. Grice, Scientific Coordinator, International Life
Sciences Institute, Nepean, Ontario, Canada

Associate Editors
Dr. Douglas L. Arnold, Bureau of Chemical Safety, Health Protection
Branch, Health and Welfare Canada, Ottawa, Ontario, Canada

Dr. David B. Clayson, Bureau of Chemical Safety, Health Protection
Branch, Health and Welfare Canada, Ottawa, Ontario, Canada

Dr. Miles D. Clarke, Bureau of Chemical Safety, Health Protection
Branch, Health and Welfare Canada, Ottawa, Ontario, Canada

Dr. John L. Emmerson, Director, Toxicology Studies, Lilly Research
Laboratories, Eli Lilly and Company, Greenfield, Indiana, U.S.A.

Dr. Lawrence Fishbein, Director, Office of Scientific Intelligence,
National Center for Toxicological Research, Jefferson,
Arkansas, U.S.A.

Dr. Donald Hughes, Scientific Coordinator, Regulatory Services
Division, The Procter and Gamble Company, Cincinnati, Ohio, U.S.A.

Dr. Daniel Krewski, Environmental Health Directorate, Health
Protection Branch, Health and Welfare Canada, Ottawa, Ontario,
Canada

Officers—ILSI

Alex Malaspina, Atlanta—President
Peter B. Dews, Boston—Vice President
Ulrich Mohr, Hannover—Vice President
Roger D. Middlekauff, Washington—Secretary/Treasurer

Contributors

R.L. Anderson, Ph.D.
The Procter and Gamble Company
Cincinnati, Ohio, U.S.A.

D.L. Arnold, Ph.D.
Health Protection Branch
Health and Welfare Canada
Ottawa, Ontario, Canada

R.G. Carlson, D.V.M., Ph.D.
Upjohn International, Inc.
Kalamazoo, Michigan, U.S.A.

C. Chang, M.D.
Department of Pediatrics
  and Human Development
Michigan State University
East Lansing, Michigan, U.S.A.

M. D. Clarke, D.V.M., M.Sc.
Health Protection Branch
Health and Welfare Canada
Ottawa, Ontario, Canada

D.B. Clayson, Ph.D.
Bureau of Chemical Safety
Health and Welfare Canada
Ottawa, Ontario, Canada

Yin Dai, Ph.D.
Institute of Health
Chinese Academy of Medical
  Science
Beijing, China

J.L. Emerson, D.V.M., Ph.D.
The Coca-Cola Company
Atlanta, Georgia, U.S.A.

L. Fishbein, Ph.D.
National Center for
  Toxicological Research
Jefferson, Arkansas, U.S.A.

S. Garattini, M.D.
Instituto di Ricerche
  Farmacologiche
Milan, Italy

H.C. Grice, D.V.M., M.Sc., V.S.
International Life Sciences Institute
Nepean, Ontario, Canada

R. Hess, M.D.
CIBA GEIGY AB
Basel, Switzerland

J.C. Kirschman, Ph.D.
General Foods Corporation
Tarrytown, New York, U.S.A.

D. Krewski, Ph.D.
Health Protection Branch
Health and Welfare Canada
Ottawa, Ontario, Canada

R. Kroes, D.V.M., Ph.D.
National Institute of Public
  Health and Environmental
  Hygiene
Bilthoven, Netherlands

C.T. Miller, Ph.D.
Priority Issues Directorate
Environment Canada
Hull, Quebec, Canada

I.C. Munro, Ph.D.
Canadian Centre for Toxicology
University of Guelph
Guelph, Ontario, Canada

P. Olsen, D.V.M., Ph.D.
National Food Institute
Soborg, Denmark

D.V. Parke, Ph.D.
Department of Biochemistry
University of Surrey
Surrey, England

J.J. Roberts, Ph.D., D.Sc.
Institute of Cancer Research
Royal Cancer Hospital
Sutton, Surrey, England

R.A. Squire, Ph.D.
The Johns Hopkins University
School of Medicine
Baltimore, Maryland, U.S.A.

J.W. Stanley, Ph.D.
PepsiCo, Inc.
Valhalla, New York, U.S.A.

J. Sugar, M.D.
Research Institute of
  Oncopathology
Budapest, Hungary

S. Takayama, M.D.
Cancer Institute
Japanese Foundation for Cancer
  Research
Tokyo, Japan

H. Tryphonas, M.Sc.
Division of Toxicology Research
Health Protection Branch
Health and Welfare Canada
Ottawa, Ontario, Canada

G.M. Williams, M.D.
Naylor Dana Institute for
  Disease Prevention
Valhalla, New York, U.S.A.

Contents

I. Introduction

The interpretation and extrapolation of animal data for predicting human health effects from carcinogens or chronic toxicants is a complex process involving many uncertainties. This document attempts to outline some of the factors involved in the process, taking into account the relevant chemical and biological properties of the compound of interest and the strengths and limitations of the test systems employed.

The toxic effects that a chemical can have on a biological system following long-term exposure are determined by the interplay of endogenous and exogenous factors. These include dose of the chemical, pharmacokinetic and metabolic interactions with cells and intracellular constituents, genetic, endocrine and immunological factors, nutritional status, and environmental influences.

Much of the basic information that is required to determine the etiology and pathogenesis of a chemically-induced toxic event is fairly well established. This includes the physical and chemical properties of the substance and its structural analogy with compounds of known activity. It also involves an assessment of the nature of clinical-pathological findings from acute, subchronic and chronic toxicity studies. Additional information includes pharmacokinetic data and reactivity of the chemical or its metabolites with macromolecules. Even though a significant amount of basic information may be available, the mechanisms of inter- and intracellular regulation involved in some types of chronic toxicological events including carcinogenesis are not fully understood.

The process of extrapolation requires an understanding of the nature and mechanisms of toxicity in animals and a subsequent assessment to determine the likelihood that such events could occur in humans. The complexities of the mechanism of action, the degree to which this can be explained or understood, and the availability of comparable human data for comparison purposes dictate to a large extent the degree to which meaningful extrapolation can be made.

One of the major problems in the extrapolation process with most chemicals is the lack of data in humans. Epidemiological results are available only for some compounds that have been present in the environment for some time and for which there is a well defined cohort of exposed individuals; these data are subject to limitations in sensitivity and to potentially confounding variables.

On occasion information concerning toxic effects of a chemical in humans may be available from reports of accidental or occupational exposure. For some widely used chemicals such as alcohol or caffeine, it is feasible to obtain data on metabolism and pharmacokinetics in man. For other chemicals, particularly those with carcinogenic potential, ethical considerations preclude the obtaining of pharmacokinetic data in humans unless the chemical is used for chemotherapy or a similar therapeutic effect. However, even when comprehensive comparative data are available, the problem of determining whether a particular effect observed in animals may also occur in humans is not a simple one, particularly if the pharmacokinetics of the chemical are different in animals and man.

When the data for extrapolation are insufficient the prudent evaluator will likely be conservative in assessing the potential risk posed to humans. In the particular area of carcinogenesis there is growing recognition of the need to distinguish between agents with different mechanisms of action and different potencies. In this document this issue is addressed by considering the spectrum of chemical and biological properties associated with animal carcinogens. A careful analysis of this information on a case-by-case basis may help to identify those animal carcinogens that may pose a greater risk to humans.

The principal source of evidence for carcinogenic potential is the chronic toxicity/carcinogenicity bioassay in rodents. A critical review of this procedure is presented in Section II, with emphasis on those features that constitute an adequate study by today's standards. The salient elements of test design, conduct and interpretation are outlined. Short-term tests which provide corroborative information are described and their predictive value is discussed in Section III. The manner in which the animal metabolizes a chemical can have a marked influence on the toxicity of the chemical. The interpretation of animal studies in the light of pharmacokinetics and metabolism is thus considered in Section IV.

If good laboratory practices are carefully adhered to in the conduct of toxicity tests, the potential for experimental animals to be exposed inadvertently to more than one toxic chemical at a time is remote. However, since humans come in contact with numerous natural and synthetic chemicals in everyday living, it is possible that they may be exposed to more than one potentially injurious chemical at any given time. Because of this there is a possibility that there will be interactions resulting in synergistic or antagonistic effects. Such effects are considered in Section V.

The key to extrapolation of carcinogenic responses in animal studies to humans lies in an understanding of the mechanisms involved in the process by which carcinogenic agents exert their effects. The present knowledge of carcinogenic mechanisms is reviewed, and the implications these carry in extrapolation to humans are considered in Section VI.

In Section VII an attempt is made to consider the various chemical and biological properties that may contribute to assessment of carcinogenic risk of chemicals to humans. The importance of considering the totality of effects of each individual chemical in making this assessment is emphasized.

The establishment of safe and realistic guidelines for human exposure to carcinogens requires the judicious utilization of all the pertinent data in defining mechanisms of toxicity. This is considered in Section VIII.

II. Chronic Toxicity/Carcinogenicity Bioassay

2.1. Introduction

Well designed and properly conducted chronic bioassays provide substantial information on the toxicity and carcinogenic potential of chemicals and mixtures of chemicals in the test animals. A long-term carcinogenicity experiment may lead to multiple end points, each of which requires careful consideration before a compound can be designated as a carcinogen or a noncarcinogen in the sex and species tested. The results of the test will be regarded as relevant if the experiment is designed in a manner which reflects the nature and use pattern of the test substance and is conducted according to accepted guidelines and practices.

There are a number of important factors that must be taken into account in the design and conduct of carcinogenicity studies in laboratory animals for the results to be meaningful for extrapolation to humans. In this section of the monograph important aspects of design, conduct and interpretation of carcinogenicity studies in laboratory animals are briefly reviewed. The following discussion is intended to define an "adequate" study and to identify the evidence of carcinogenicity in animal studies.

2.2. Identity, Analytical Purity and Stability of Test Substances

There is increasing recognition that in any meaningful evaluation of biological and toxicological data, it is vital that particular attention be addressed to considerations of the physical and chemical properties of the test chemicals, the purity and the nature of the impurities, as well as the reactivity and stability of both parent compound and impurities under conditions of storage or administration (Bowman, 1969; Burchfield *et al.*, 1977; Coleman and Tardiff, 1979; de Serres and Ashby, 1981a; FSC, 1978; IARC, 1972-1980; Munro, 1977; NAS, 1975; Page, 1977; WHO, 1978). The value of any study will be greatly enhanced by precise knowledge of the chemical structure and purity of the test substance and of the nature and amount of impurities present. It is general practice in toxicological studies to rely on tests involving either purified chemical substances or commercial products to which humans are exposed, recognizing that the latter material may contain a number of impurities of possibly unknown toxic potential.

The stability of the substance should be determined under actual conditions of storage and use in order to prescribe the manner in which the chemical should be stored *per se* or in appropriate dosage vehicles to prevent decomposition.

Detailed knowledge of the chemical reactivity of a substance is essential, particularly in feeding studies where the test agent may react with the constituents present in the laboratory diet or dosing vehicle. For example, chemical binding or absorption by macromolecules in the diet may appreciably alter the rate and extent of absorption of the agent from the gastrointestinal tract, or reactive groups of the test substance may be neutralized by dietary constituents. Conversely, reaction of the test substance with essential dietary constituents may contribute to nutritional deficiency states or the formation of more toxic compounds (Jones *et al.*, 1971).

The vapor pressure of volatile test substances is of obvious importance, particularly in inhalation studies which are influenced by the extent to which a solid or liquid vaporizes under controlled conditions (Jones *et al.*, 1971). In the design of inhalation studies, knowledge of the toxicity of aerosols, including their particle size, shape and density is important since these factors are prerequisites for the determination of the site of deposition and the rates and mechanism for clearance from the respiratory tract (Hatch and Gross, 1964). Animals fed diets containing volatile materials will be subject to exposure by the inhalation route and a diminished exposure by the oral route. Knowledge of the mode of administration and the quantities ingested is essential for proper interpretation of the findings in the study. The particle size of substances administered orally via suspensions can markedly influence their absorption (WHO, 1978).

2.3. Species and Strain of Test Animals

Virtually all studies designed to evaluate carcinogenic potential employ rats, mice or Syrian hamsters. These animals are used extensively because (a) their natural life span is short; (b) it is practical to breed, maintain and handle them in large numbers; (c) they are relatively inexpensive to purchase and maintain; (d) strains can be obtained that are genetically homogeneous and therefore respond with some uniformity in the spontaneous incidence of cancer, in susceptibility to carcinogens at specific organ sites, in longevity, and in response to husbandry systems; (e) these species have been shown to be responsive to treatment by most known human carcinogens (IARC, 1979a); and (f) there is a large historical data base of the carcinogenic responses to various chemicals by rats and mice and the incidence of various types of spontaneous tumors in these species. A knowledge of the normal background incidence of spontaneous diseases and tumors by type and system in any colony under standardized conditions is necessary for the proper evaluation of experimental findings in a bioassay. It is also important to recognize that a specific strain of rodent may vary from one supplier to another in the incidence of spontaneous tumors and disease. There is no good scientific rationale to recommend either inbred, outbred, hybrid, or randombred strains (Health Council of the Netherlands, 1980; IARC, 1980b; OECD, 1981). It is acknowledged that the use of these animal species is based more on cost and the ease of conduct of the experiment than on biochemical, physiological or anatomical similarities to man. Ideally, the particular species selected should be a physiological model for man producing the same spectrum of metabolites and similar concentrations of the chemical and/or metabolites at the target tissue, and responding to treatment in a fashion analogous to man.

2.4. Route of Administration

As a general rule, the route of administration should approximate as closely as possible the expected route of exposure in man. However, a different route of exposure may be used in certain cases if there are sufficient data demonstrating that equivalent tissue levels of the test material and metabolites may be obtained from an alternate route of exposure. It is essential that the pharmacokinetics for each chemical be assessed with respect to the route of administration selected.

2.5. Dose Selection and Treatment Groups

The selection of the number of treatment groups and corresponding doses in chronic toxicity/carcinogenicity studies is dealt with in detail elsewhere (Grice and Burek, 1983). The general principles involved in the selection

of doses, taking into account both the development of the study protocol
and factors involved in the interpretation of the results, are considered in
the document. It is important that the selection of doses to be used is based
on information that will maximize the likelihood that any induced effects
are relevant to the safety assessment process. The rationale for dose
selection should be outlined in the study report to allow for proper
evaluation of the study results.

2.6. Sample Size

In general, a sufficient number of animals should be allocated to each test
group in order to ensure adequate statistical sensitivity. It has become
standard practice to use at least 50 animals of each sex per group in long-
term carcinogenicity studies. While groups of five or ten animals will serve
for the detection of potent carcinogens, groups of 50 animals provide an
acceptable level of conviction when negative results are obtained.
Experiments involving 50 animals may be expected to detect effects
involving about 10% or more of the target population with a fair degree of
certainty (Krewski et al., 1982). If interim sacrifices are to be taken, then
an additional number of animals should be predesignated for this purpose.
Such sacrifices are useful in the evaluation of the progressive pathogenesis
of the lesions present and provide a better data base for time-adjusted
statistical analyses (see Section 2.14).

2.7. Methods of Randomization

The importance of proper randomization in experimental design cannot be
overemphasized (Mantel, 1980); careful analyses of carcinogenicity
studies have revealed possible cage and rack effects as well as litter effects
on tumor production (Lagakos and Mosteller, 1981).

    One approach would be to randomize completely: animals to cages and
cages to treatments. Although reasonable in statistical terms, such a
design may result in diet cross-contamination due to either technician
error, spillage of the feed or volatility of the test compound. In such cases,
clustered designs in which contiguous cages are treated alike may be
considered, although the statistical analysis may have to be modified
accordingly (Bickis and Krewski, 1984). Complete randomization may
not always be the most appropriate design if one wishes to exploit possible
intra-litter correlation. By stratification within litters (i.e., randomization
of littermates to different treatment groups) the statistical sensitivity of the
study may be enhanced. Stratification may involve other extraneous

factors such as cagemates or cage location (Fox *et al.*, 1979). In multi-generation studies, randomization within litters is not possible, thus the litter should be considered the experimental unit for analysis purposes (Haseman and Kupper, 1979).

Unfortunately, it is not possible to prescribe the best randomization procedure to be followed in all cases. Nonetheless, experiments should be carefully planned with the foreknowledge that the outcome may be severely compromised due to lack of randomization. From the operational point of view, care must be taken to ensure that the desired dose is in fact delivered to the designated animals with a minimum of error.

2.8. Duration of Studies

It has become common practice in long-term carcinogenicity studies to dose mice and rats with the test chemical from shortly after weaning throughout the major portion of their lifespan. Eighteen and 24-month periods have been used for mice and rats, respectively, because survival rates fall markedly after that time. However, the availability of healthier stocks that are resistant to many of the enzootic diseases common in earlier investigations, together with improved animal care, has resulted in better survival rates. This has led to proposals that the duration of chronic studies should be extended beyond the 18 to 24-month period. The Interagency Regulatory Liaison Group (IRLG, 1979) reports that "the best negative evidence for the carcinogenicity of a substance is obtained from tests in which both exposure and observation last through all or nearly all of the expected life span of the animals under study." While this statement may be true, conducting studies of these durations is difficult in practice and probably unnecessary for the reasons outlined below. The International Agency for Research on Cancer (IARC, 1980b) suggests that:

> the following procedures might be an acceptable compromise: the survivors in all groups are killed and the whole experiment is terminated if the mortality in the control or low dose group ever reaches 75%. However, in any case, the study is not continued beyond week 130 of age for rats, 120 for mice and 100 weeks for hamsters, irrespective of mortality. Except for studies in which the cause of death was from tumors that were induced, an experiment is not really a satisfactory long-term carcinogenicity study if the mortality in the control or low dose group is higher than 50% before the end of week 104 of age of rats, week 96 for mice and week 80 for hamsters. With respect to termination, the males and females are treated as separate experiments.

The duration of toxicity studies is dealt with in detail in the International Life Sciences Institute (ILSI) monograph on geriatric pathology (Grice and Burek, 1983). In determining the duration of a study, two major principles should be considered. The first is concerned with the increasing prevalence of naturally occurring disease processes in aging animals at about two years and beyond (Goodman *et al.*, 1980). The use of unhealthy animals is contrary to a basic requirement in toxicity studies and must be avoided. The second principle relates to the fact that evidence of chemically-induced carcinogenicity will likely be apparent in rodents prior to 24 months in appropriately designed and conducted studies (Grice and Burek, 1983). These realities strongly suggest that a fixed point for the termination of the study (e.g., 24 months in rats) is preferable. The issue of lifespan or two-year studies for carcinogen testing was considered by Solleveld *et al.* (1983). They noted that the variety of lesions was not greater in animals of the lifespan study than in those of two-year studies; and increasing age is not characterized by unique neoplasms. The incidence of certain neoplasms in control animals increased markedly after 110-116 weeks of age. They conclude that for the F 344 rat, lifespan studies in general have no advantage over two-year studies in carcinogenicity investigations.

The protocol should be sufficiently flexible to allow for extension of studies beyond the specified period. For example, if a particular tumor type appears to be occurring with increasing frequency late in the course of the study, it might be desirable to extend the study.

2.9. Clinical Observations

One of the most critical aspects of a carcinogenicity study is the conduct of clinical examinations of the animal during the test period. Much useful information can be derived from such data, as long as consistent criteria are used in documenting the observations taken (Arnold *et al.*, 1978; Fox *et al.*, 1979; IARC, 1980b). In-life phase observations form the basis for time-to-tumor calculations and are essential for a complete understanding of onset and progression of chronic toxicoses.

2.10. Animal Husbandry

Animal husbandry practices can greatly influence the outcome and eventual value of a carcinogenesis study and are therefore as important as any other part of the experimental protocol. As in any experimental situation it is important to eliminate the potential confounding effects of as many extraneous environmental factors as possible. Thus, factors such as temperature, air flow, illumination, and humidity should be held constant throughout the experiment (Fox, 1977).

2.11. Diet

Food consumption can be an important factor in the outcome of a carcinogenesis study because caloric intake and other factors of dietary composition can influence tumor yield (Tannenbaum, 1944, 1949; Tucker, 1979). Caloric restriction is capable of decreasing the incidence of spontaneous or induced tumors. This would be the net result, for example, if an added substance rendered a diet less palatable to the test animal. It is therefore important to ascertain any such effect in a pilot study prior to undertaking a carcinogenesis study. High fat diets are associated with a high incidence of breast cancer in humans and laboratory animals (Carroll, 1980; Rogers, 1983). Protein-deficient rats are highly susceptible to the acute toxic effects of aflatoxin B1, yet they are relatively resistant to its carcinogenicity (Madhaven and Gopalan, 1968; Rogers and Newberne, 1971). The quality of dietary protein and the levels of dietary essentials such as tryptophan, riboflavin and methionine may also influence tumor incidence (Rogers and Newberne, 1971; Rogers, 1975; Shinozuka et al., 1978). High doses of the test material can also compromise the nutritional adequacy of the basal diet throughout. It is important, therefore, to use a diet that is consistent in quality and nutritionally complete for the species of animal used. Those constituents that could interfere with the outcome of the study such as toxic fungal products, antioxidants, heavy metals, and pesticides should certainly be minimized in any diet to the greatest extent possible (Bowman, 1969; Coleman and Tardif, 1979; Edwards et al., 1979; Fishbein, 1979). The potential of the test compound to compromise the nutritional adequacy (i.e., by dilution or feed refusal) of the diet should also be carefully evaluated. The use of semisynthetic purified diets has been recommended as a means of controlling the above problems, but these diets are not problem-free and except in special circumstances their use cannot be generally recommended. Open formula diets made from natural foodstuffs are now commercially available. As they are of reasonably constant composition, they are preferable for routine carcinogenesis studies. Care should be taken that these diets are properly stored, considering time and temperature, until fed to the test animals. The constituents of open formula diets are reported and may be preferable to closed formula diets where the formulas are not reported.

2.12. Pathology

It is very important that a proper gross examination is carried out on all animals at the time of necropsy (Health Council of the Netherlands, 1980;

IRLG, 1979; WHO, 1978). Prior to the gross examination, it is essential to review the clinical history of the animal. Care must be taken to note and identify all gross observations and document any discrepancies between the clinical history and gross findings. This is facilitated by the use of appropriately trained and experienced prosectors under the supervision of a pathologist experienced in the species used.

Examination of animals dying or killed during the course of a study may provide information that will prompt a change in the protocol for the rest of the study period. Such measures may provide data important to final interpretation of the results, e.g., hematology from animals dying of chemically-induced blood dyscrasias.

A pathologist skilled in the species used should initially screen all tissues collected from animals of the high dose and control groups. The decision to perform histological evaluation of the animals in low and middle dose groups depends upon the evaluation of the gross necropsy findings and the results of histopathologic examination of the control and high dose group.

Animals that have died or were killed in a moribund state should be histologically examined prior to the end of the study. In some cases these animals may provide early information regarding the potential toxicity and/or carcinogenicity of a substance. Information obtained early in the course of the study on the pathogenesis of induced lesions allows for special attention to be paid to particular organs. It also aids in determining if the study should be extended beyond the period specified in the protocol. It is essential in performing histological examinations that all gross lesions are histologically examined and that all relevant clinical information is available at the time of examination. This can only be ensured by careful checking and correlation of all gross, hematologic, serum, chemical and microscopic findings.

In recording microscopic lesions, a systematic and standard format should be used to ensure examination of all tissues in a consistent manner. Hyperplastic and neoplastic lesions should be tabulated by organ system. Consideration must be given to the following on an organ or system basis:

a. total number of animals examined;
b. total number of tissues examined;
c. total number of animals with benign or malignant tumors of specified types;
d. tumor multiplicity of specified types for individual animals;
e. total number of hyperplastic lesions associated with various tumor types.

In order that time-adjusted analyses may be performed, it is important that the survival time of each animal also be recorded. Any information on the possible cause of death or contributing factors should also be noted.

2.13. Factors That May Modulate Tumor Occurrence

When there is an increase in the incidence of a particular tumor type over the background incidence, it is necessary to determine if factors other than the test chemical may have caused or contributed to the increased incidence. A first step in this process is to compare tumor incidence of treated animals with that of concurrent and, if necessary, historical control animals. It is known that inter- and intra-laboratory variability in control incidence frequently exceeds what could be expected to be found by chance alone (Flamm, 1983; Haseman, 1983; Tarone *et al.*, 1981). There are various factors that are known to alter tumor incidence in laboratory animals, including the microbiological status of the test animals, various forms of stress, immune modulation, hormonal status, diurnal rhythms and disease processes such as ocular lesions. The following section is devoted to a consideration of these factors.

Microbiological Status of Test Animals. The microbiological status of test animals can influence the outcome and the evaluation of toxicity studies. Prior to modern methods of commercial animal rearing and the maintenance of test animals in adequate facilities, the most common reason for invalidating studies was the fact that the vast majority of the animals died prematurely from infectious diseases. Gart *et al.* (1979) have considered how mortality from infectious disease may introduce competing risk prejudicial to the accurate statistical analysis of tumor incidence. Hanna *et al.* (1973) have shown that variance in the microbiologic status of control groups may be responsible for variation in historical control tumor incidence data in some instances. Roe and Grant (1970) found that germ-free male C_3H mice develop significantly fewer mouse hepatocellular tumors following the neonatal administration of 7,12-dimethylbenz(a)anthracene. Mizutani and Mitsuoka (1979) found that the spontaneous incidence of mouse hepatocellular neoplasia was higher in conventionalized mice derived from germ-free mice, and also in gnotobiotes infected with a specific strain of bacteria which then populated the colon.

Viral oncogenesis in rats and mice tends to occur in well-defined, planned situations and is probably not a major complicating factor in most carcinogenesis bioassays. A recent finding (Rizzino *et al.*, 1982) which warrants attention is the recovery of a retrovirus apparently capable of causing pulmonary alveologenic adenocarcinoma in mice.

There are a number of reports concerned with interactions between chemicals and viruses in the process of oncogenesis. Several reports (Fish *et al.*, 1981; Weislow *et al.*, 1978; Whitmire, 1973; Whitmire and Salerno, 1973) have dealt with the somewhat complex interactions between retroviruses and 3-methylcholanthrene in induction of leukemias and sarcomas in rats and mice. Retroviruses are known to inhibit development of some transplanted tumors in mice (Kelloff *et al.*, 1976). Hamsters innoculated with parvovirus H-1 were refractory to induction of tumors by 7,12-dimethylbenz(a)anthracene (Toolan *et al.*, 1982). Sendai virus in mice apparently can affect induction of lung adenomas by urethane (Parker and Richter, 1982). Chemically-induced mouse lung tumorigenesis has been suppressed by concurrent infection with murine sarcoma virus (Stoner *et al.*, 1974), reovirus (Theiss *et al.*, 1978), and lactate dehydrogenase virus (Theiss *et al.*, 1980). All of these effects were attributed to augmentation of the immune response to the neoplasm. Prehn (1973) showed that tumor cell destruction can be augmented by non-specific factors activated by a specific immunologic reaction against antigens unrelated to those of the tumor cells.

Respiratory mycoplasmosis in rats has been shown to have been a permissive factor in the development of pulmonary squamous cell carcinomas induced by N-nitrosoheptamethyleneimine (Schreiber *et al.*, 1972).

Modification of immune function (particularly cell-mediated immunity) can occur as a result of infections with Sendai virus (Garlinghouse and Van Hoosier, 1978; Kay *et al.*, 1979), lactate dehydrogenase-elevating virus (Howard *et al.*, 1969; Riley *et al.*, 1978), cytomegalovirus (Selgrade *et al.*, 1976), and lymphocytic choriomeningitis virus (Bro-Jorgensen *et al.*, 1975; Lohler and Lehmann, 1979). Lymphocytic choriomeningitis virus augments natural killer cell activity in mice (Welsh, 1978; Welsh *et al.*, 1979). Sendai virus has also been shown to enhance anti-tumor cytotoxicity in mice (Clark *et al.*, 1979; Takeyama *et al.*, 1979).

Interferon, the synthesis of which is known to be induced by viral replication, has been shown to exert an inhibitory effect on both spontaneous (De Clerca *et al.*, 1982) and chemically-induced (Salerno *et al.*, 1972) tumors in mice. Direct virus-induced synthesis and release of corticosterone by the adrenal cortex, possibly mediated through interferon and lymphocytes, has recently been proposed as an additional "sensory" mechanism eliciting glucocorticoid biosynthesis (Smith *et al.*, 1982).

Stress. Stresses of perception (social conditions, restraint, handling, noise, fighting, cold, electric shock) or what Newberry (1981) calls "presumably stressful stimulation" (PSS) have been examined by a number of laboratories for their effects on tumor transplantability, and to a lesser extent on spontaneous, viral, and chemically-induced tumorigenesis (Amkraut and Solomon, 1972; Riley, 1975, 1981; Sklar and Anisman, 1980, 1981). The available data support the idea of chronic stress as a modifying factor in the post-initiation development of clones of initiated cells.

Several papers (Sklar and Anisman, 1979; Visintainer *et al.*, 1982) relate higher growth rates or lower rejection rates of transplantable tumors to inescapable, as opposed to escapable electric shock. Depletion of hypothalamic and cerebral norepinephrine has been associated with inescapable as opposed to escapable stress (Anisman *et al.*, 1980; Weiss *et al.*, 1975). Sklar and Anisman (1981) regard brain catecholamine metabolism as pivotal in the mediation of social and physical stress on tumor growth. Activation of the hypothalamic-adenohypophyseal-adrenal cortical axis is involved in depressing the immune reactivity of the animal (Amkraut and Solomon, 1972; Riley, 1981).

Within-laboratory and between-laboratory heterogeneity in control tumor data, as was observed by Tarone *et al.* (1981), could arise as a result of such factors as differing degrees of skill in animal palpation by technicians.

Immune Function. The immune system is a highly complex network of cellular components which interact in a tightly regulated manner (Bier *et al.*, 1981). These cellular components are under a dynamic process of proliferation and differentiation. Consequently, an imbalance in this regulatory network brought about by chemical treatment will ultimately be expressed as an immune alteration. The latter may be expressed either as immune enhancement which often results in autoimmunity, allergy, or contact hypersensitivity, or as immune suppression, which may lead to decreased resistance to infection or may impair the host's defenses against a neoplastic process. The precise mechanisms by which neoplastic cells escape the host's immune processes are not well understood.

Recent advances in immunology, however, have provided new and promising tools for further elucidating such a mechanism. For example, the various cell types of the immune system can now be segregated and purified by flow cytometry techniques and their functions can be assessed *in vitro* by the use of monoclonal antibodies. As a result, several *in vivo* and *in vitro* immunoassays are available and are used to study the possible involvement of the immune system in the development of malignancy following chemical exposure to laboratory animals.

Prior to initiating studies of this kind, however, it is advisable to examine carefully data from short-term toxicity studies for possible clues to any immune alterations. In this respect, body weight/organ weight ratios, routinely determined in toxicologic studies, are useful indicators of organ toxicity.

Since immune suppression may be either secondary to generalized toxicity, or a direct immunotoxic effect of the chemical, it is important that the investigator incorporates histopathologic studies of the lymphoid organs in the initial design of the experiment. Morphological evaluation of these organs, when combined with morphometric techniques, may suggest which component of the immune system is being affected. Thymic atrophy, for example, has been observed following exposure to many chemicals and appears to be an extremely sensitive indicator of chemical immunotoxicity, correlating well with cell-mediated immune (CMI) aberrations (Dean *et al.*, 1982). However, this parameter alone should not be considered as a specific indicator of direct chemically-induced immunotoxicity, since it is known that stress and general toxicity can also result in thymic atrophy (Keller, 1983). Consequently, histopathological examination, especially of the thymic cortical elements which contain lymphocytes that are not fully immunocompetent (immature T-cells), is of significance in determining the site of chemical immunotoxicity.

Similarly, histopathological studies are recommended for lymphoid organs including bone marrow, spleen and lymph nodes (mesenteric and peripheral). Histologic evaluation of the spleen, for example, combined with hematologic examination may provide helpful information in determining the nature of an observed weight change in this organ. A reduction in the size of the splenic lymphoid follicles at the germinal centers would be indicative of B-lymphocyte deficiency, while lymphoid hypoplasia in the paracortical areas would be characteristic of T-cell deficiency (Bier *et al.*, 1981).

If an effect of the chemical on the immune system is observed, it would be desirable to determine if this effect played any role in the health status of the animal, and particularly in tumor development. If such studies are undertaken, *in vivo* and *in vitro* immunoassays should be selected to test all components of the immune system including the bone marrow, cellular and humoral immunity and macrophage function. The selection of a wide range of assays is important in relation to chemical carcinogenesis since it has been shown in recent years that immune surveillance against neoplasia includes not only thymus-dependent CMI responses (Burnet, 1970) but other non-cell-mediated immune components and factors (Evans, 1983). For example, activated peritoneal macrophages from nude (athymic) mice have been shown to possess tumoricidal activity (Meltzer, 1976), and a non T-lymphocyte-dependent resistance to polyoma oncogenesis has been described in nude mice (Warner *et al.*, 1977). Recently, a category of lymphocytes has been characterized which appears to have cytotoxic activity against neoplastic cells in the absence of prior sensitization (Herberman and Holden, 1978; Herberman and Ortaldo, 1981; Riccardi *et al.*, 1980). A deficiency of these "natural killer" (NK) cells is associated with increased tumor susceptibility in beige mice (Karre *et al.*, 1980; Talmadge *et al.*, 1980). NK cells may be either activated or suppressed by a number of factors (Evans *et al.*, 1982; Hisano and Hanna, 1982), particularly by suppressor cells (Broder *et al.*, 1978; Schechter and Feldman, 1979), and prostaglandins (Alexander, 1982; Brunda *et al.*, 1980). Suppression of NK cell cytotoxicity, resulting from certain forms of stress, has been shown to be mediated by endogenous opioid peptides (Shavit *et al.*, 1984). Oral administration of dimethylbenzanthracene to mice caused a marked and lasting decline in the splenic NK cell activity (Ehrlich *et al.*, 1983). In studies with 3-methylcholanthrene, Kalland and Forsberg (1983) suggest that a possible part of the tumorigenic effect of 3-methylcholanthrene is its early suppressive effect on NK cell activity. Cox *et al.* (1983) have shown that the production of NK cytotoxicity factors in tumor cell-stimulated nude mouse spleen cell culture was severely depressed after glucocorticoid treatment. This suggests that a stressed animal may have a diminished capacity for immune surveillance against incipient tumor cell clones. NK cells also play an important role in the destruction of circulating tumor emboli (Gorelik *et al.*, 1982; Hanna and Fidler, 1980; Lundy *et al.*, 1977).

Recent papers (Gorelik and Herberman, 1981a, 1981b) have demonstrated that the susceptibility of various mouse strains to urethane induction of lung adenomas is proportional to the degree of suppression by urethane of NK cells, the presence of which has been demonstrated in mouse lung (Puccetti *et al.*, 1980; Riccardi *et al.*, 1979). From an immunologic standpoint it is conceivable that an increase in mouse lung tumors might be ascribed to a permissive effect of treatment.

A proposed battery of functional *in vivo* and *in vitro* immunoassays has been described in detail elsewhere (Dean *et al.*, 1982). These assays are grouped for practical purposes under the general headings of cell-mediated immunity, humoral immunity (HI) and macrophage function. It would seem appropriate to undertake immune function tests when and if evidence of immune system effects arose in the subchronic and chronic studies and further elucidation of the mechanisms involved was desired.

In vivo assays used frequently to test competence of CMI include: delayed-type hypersensitivity, graft vs. host reactions, and rejection of skin grafts. *In vitro* techniques include: lymphokine production, T-cell cytotoxicity, and lymphoproliferative assays using specific antigens or the polyclonal mitogens phytohemagglutinin, concanavallin A, and *Escherichia coli* lipopolysaccharide.

HI in chemically-treated animals is most appropriately determined by enumerating antibody plaque-forming cell numbers, antibody production to T-cell dependent antigens (e.g., sheep red blood cells), and T-cell independent or B-cell dependent antigens (e.g., *Escherichia coli* lipopolysaccharide). Determination of serum immunoglobulin concentrations is especially useful in chronic studies where sufficient time is available for the gradual degradation of existing (pre-exposure) immunoglobulin levels.

Procedures also exist to assess the functional properties of macrophages. Macrophages can be easily enumerated by staining for non-specific esterase activity. Methods have also been established to test for *in vitro* phagocytosis of inert particles, intracellular killing, and cytostasis/cytolysis of virally-infected or transformed cells. Enumeration of live residual bacteria in the spleen and liver of experimental and control animals over a period of time has proven to be a useful indicator of the body's defense capability against infection.

The various immunoassays mentioned in this section may be applied to the quantitative and functional assessment of generalized immune processes. However, in recent years evidence has been presented to suggest that immunity as defined by these assays does not always reflect events at the tumor site. Various immune effectors may be selectively prevented from reaching the tumor site because of structural or chemical barriers. Similarly a selected subpopulation of immune effector components at the tumor site may have a completely different biological effect from those generated by the more heterogeneous population of peripheral immune components.

Recent methodological advances (Witz and Hanna, 1980) have included procedures from the isolation, identification, and functional assessment of tumor-derived immune components. Hence a comprehensive understanding of immune function and its relation to chemical carcinogenesis would require a detailed analysis of the *in situ* tumor immunity as well as that of effector mechanisms operating elsewhere in the body.

Hormonal Status. The mechanism(s) by which hormones influence cancer development is not understood. A list of possible mechanisms has been proposed (IARC, 1979b) which includes increased binding of chemical carcinogens to cellular constituents, the activation of oncogenic virus production, immunosuppression, formation of preneoplastic cells, preferential stimulation of abnormal cell populations, stimulation of DNA synthesis and mitosis, and hormonal imbalance which may favor proliferation over functional differentiation. Neither the hormones nor any of their metabolic products have been shown convincingly to be mutagenic (IARC, 1983). However, there have been reports of covalent binding of diethylstilbestrol metabolites to DNA, and of results in short-term tests that indicated interactions with DNA (IARC, 1983; Martin et al., 1978). Hormonal effects on the incidence of mouse hepatocellular neoplasia are well recognized. The incidence of such lesions in male mice is slightly to markedly higher than in females (Grasso and Hardy, 1975). Castration of male C_3H mice reduced the incidence of hepatocellular neoplasms by a third (Andervont, 1950). Agnew and Gardner (1952) reported that the incidence of hepatic neoplasms was increased in female C_3H mice treated with testosterone. Synthetic and natural female sex hormones are promoting agents in liver carcinogenesis in the rat (Cameron et al., 1982; Goldfarb, 1976; Yager and Yager, 1980).

There appears to be a relationship between prolactin and mammary tumorigenesis in the rat (Mori et al., 1980; Welsch and Nagasawa, 1977; Welsch and DeHoog, 1983). The influence of exogenous prolactin on 7,12-dimethylbenz(a)anthracene (DMBA)-induced mammary tumors is critically affected by the sequence of prolactin and DMBA administration. The stimulatory effect of prolactin on the growth of rat mammary tumors induced by N-nitroso-N-methylurea is less than on tumors induced by DMBA (Gandilhon et al., 1983). Initiation, as well as promotion, of rat mammary tumors by prolactin has been suggested (Welsch and Nagasawa, 1977). The promotional effect of prolactin has been used to manifest clones of neoplastic mammary gland cells initiated in rats by low doses of N-nitroso-N-butylurea (Yokoro et al., 1977). Studies by Sylvester et al. (1983) suggest that rats made deficient in estrogen and prolactin at the time of DMBA administration develop fewer tumors, but the tumors that develop are not dependent on these hormones for subsequent development.

A somewhat less clear-cut relationship appears to exist between thyroid follicular cell tumors and endogenous secretion of thyrotropin by the adenohypophysis in the rat (Napalkov, 1976).

Epidemiological evidence has implicated hormones in the etiology of human ovarian cancer (Hamilton et al., 1983a) in that there is an increased incidence of the disease at or near the climateric. The existence of steroid hormone receptors in fresh epithelial ovarian tumors has been reported (Berqquist et al., 1981; Galli et al., 1981; Hamilton et al., 1982; Hamilton et al., 1983a; Schwartz et al., 1982).

Hamilton et al. (1983b) established a cell line from a patient with adenocarcinoma of the ovary which was transplantable to athymic mice.

The cultured cells and xenographs contained cytoplasmic androgen and estrogen binding macromolecules with the specificity of the respective steroid hormone receptors. Such systems should prove useful in investigating the significance of androgens and estrogens in the genesis of ovarian cancer.

Ocular Lesions. Excessive light intensities in the animal colony can cause retinal lesions in rats (Anderson *et al.*, 1972; Grignolo *et al.*, 1969; Noell *et al.*, 1966; Noell and Albrecht, 1971; O'Steen *et al.*, 1974; Reiter and Klein, 1971) and in mice (Robison and Kuwabara, 1976). The progress of this phototoxic retinopathy is accelerated in rats (Bellhorn, 1980; Weisse *et al.*, 1974) and in mice (Greenman *et al.*, 1982) by proximity to the light source, i.e., by location of the animal at the top rather than at the bottom of the cage rack. Pharmacologically or environmentally-induced increases in body temperature enhance phototoxic retinopathy in rats (Noell *et al.*, 1966). A mydriatic drug, clonidine, (Weisse *et al.*, 1971) accelerated the onset of phototoxic retinopathy in rats. A number of other compounds, including morphine (Wallenstein, 1981) and tetrahydrocannabinol (Korczyn and Eshel, 1982) have mydriatic effects in the rat and could presumably contribute to the development of phototoxic retinopathy.

Direct toxic effects upon the retina of the rat have been demonstrated with 2-aminooxypropionic acid derivatives (Lee *et al.*, 1979), chloroquine (Abraham and Hendy, 1970), urethane (Kritzinger and Bellhorn, 1982), and hexachlorophene (Rose *et al.*, 1981).

Infectious disease, such as sialodacryoadenitis virus infection in rats (Lai *et al.*, 1976; Weisbroth and Peress, 1977) and lymphocytic choriomeningitis virus infection in neonatal rats (del Cerro *et al.*, 1982) can cause significant ocular damage.

Any effects on the retina are of importance because it is known that light levels and character can influence tumor incidence and progression in rats (Hamilton, 1969) and in mice (Chignell *et al.*, 1981). This effect is thought to be mediated through the pineal gland and its secretory product, melatonin (Cardinali, 1981; Wurtman and Moskowitz, 1977).

Diurnal Rhythms. The basal activities of several drug-metabolizing enzymes in rat liver undergo circadian oscillations, with night values generally 20-30% greater than the mean (Chedid and Nair, 1971; Radzialowski and Bosquet, 1968; Schevins *et al.*, 1974). Phenobarbital sleeping times in the rat are longer during the day than at night (Schevins *et al.*, 1974). A nocturnal peak in hepatocellular smooth endoplasmic reticulum volume has been documented in the rat (Chedid and Nair, 1971). Factors which influence hepatocellular metabolic activities have the potential to influence tumor incidence. Whether or not the effects associated with diurnal rhythms have any practical consequence with respect to carcinogenicity bioassays has yet to be established.

From the foregoing it is apparent that numerous variables may modulate the tumor incidence. There is a need for a better understanding of how these factors result in altered incidences and how they might interact in modifying a carcinogenic response.

2.14. Statistical Analysis

An important interpretive aspect in carcinogenicity studies is the statistical evaluation of the data. In theory it should be possible to formulate a set of statistical decision rules designed to meet some criteria of optimality with respect to false positive and false negative error rates. In practice, however, the complex problems of numerous correlated multiple comparisons have led to the use of statistics as an aid in the decision making process rather than as an automatic decision making tool (Gart et al., 1979).

There has recently been much discussion on the effects of differences in mortality rates on the statistical comparison of tumors observed in treatment and control groups (Peto et al., 1980). Statistical methods are now available for comparing tumor rates between groups after adjusting for mortality differences. These methods must be used very carefully, since they can lead to serious biases in the comparisons. If, for instance, early mortality occurs in a treated group, then the existing prevalence of nonlethal tumors may be considered overestimated, unless corrections can be made regarding cause of death. In general, mortality corrections are likely to be most reliable whenever the tumor is either nearly always fatal or almost never fatal. The cases that fall between may require accurate information on the cause of death for proper resolution (Kodell et al., 1982).

As an aid in interpreting the significance of observed tumor patterns, comparisons with historical control rates have been proposed (Society of Toxicology, 1981). If statistical methods are used to compare data to historical controls, then the historical control data must be evaluated to determine whether the historical variation could be due to binomial variability within a single population, or whether there appears to be differences between historical control values (Dempster et al., 1983; Hoel, 1983; Tarone, 1982).

2.15. Perinatal Exposure—*In Utero* Exposure

In addition to extending studies to cover a greater period of the animal's lifetime, toxicologists are considering the need to include perinatal exposed animals in chronic toxicity studies (Grice *et al.*, 1980). When an *in utero* exposure study is employed, the test chemical may pass through several maternal and fetal tissues in addition to those tissues and organs it passes through in the non-pregnant female. These tissues have the potential to alter the chemical so that it is more or less toxic than the parent compound. The chemical or its metabolites have the potential to act on developing tissues that may be more or less susceptible to toxic effects than is the mature tissue. Furthermore, when material is administered in the diet or in the drinking water at a fixed concentration, it is important to recognize that the maternal animal's intake of the test chemical will be increased during pregnancy. Thus, metabolic and pharmacokinetic data are as essential in the design of *in utero* studies as in the interpretation of the study results.

2.16. Interpretation of Results

Long-term carcinogenicity experiments yield a spectrum of data which requires definitive consideration before a compound can be designated a carcinogen or a noncarcinogen for the test animal. In such considerations, it is important to define "carcinogen" and to realize that carcinogens may not always have the same mechanism of action and that carcinogens vary in their potency. (See Section 7.1 for definition of a carcinogen.)

The results of a long-term carcinogenicity test will be regarded as relevant for risk assessment purposes if the experiment is planned and performed in a manner which reflects the nature and intended use pattern of the test substance(s), and if the studies are designed and conducted according to internationally accepted guidelines.

The evidence of carcinogenicity for a given study is more conclusive when there are (is):

- positive results in several treated groups in a multidose study;
- positive results in a dose-related trend;
- induction of tumors exhibiting malignant biological behavior;
- positive results as reflected by a spectrum of precursor lesions, e.g., hyperplasia or benign neoplasia as well as malignant tumors;
- induction of primarily rare malignant tumor types;
- a shift of benign to malignant tumors within the same tissue;

- increased tumor incidence in tissues of different histogenetic origin (i.e., tumors derived from different embryonic germ layers, which would most often be expressed as carcinomas and sarcomas);
- decreased latency and increased total incidence of spontaneous malignant tumor types;
- multiple tumors of a particular type occurring in the same tissue;
- increased incidence of a particular tumor type in both sexes.

The value of each of the effects described above in determining the nature of carcinogenic activity of a substance is not identical and the results must be carefully evaluated in each case. Caution should be used in assessing such enhanced tumor incidences.

As more data become available from studies conducted according to good laboratory practice (GLP) and on which there is good survival to 24 months, it is apparent that some of the common tumors of rodents often show significantly different incidences between control groups (Flamm, 1983; Haseman, 1983; Tarone et al., 1981; Task Force of Past Presidents, 1982). Because of this, the Task Force of Past Presidents considered in some detail the need to take historical data into consideration. They identified several propositions that may be taken as scientifically useful in the evaluation of a chemical carcinogenic response. They drew distinctions between the use of concurrent control and historical data.

The fact that significant differences in tumor incidence can occur between control groups demonstrates the danger of considering animal studies in isolation, and the need to look beyond the particular animal study in attempting to determine whether there is biological relevance in the statistical observation.

Squire (1981a, 1981b) has proposed a system for ranking animal carcinogens that takes into account the most relevant toxicological evidence derived from animal studies. Proposals such as this are a useful starting point in assigning levels of concern to individual animal studies.

2.17. Predictive Value of Chronic Toxicity/Carcinogenicity Bioassays

In the past, the chronic toxicity/carcinogenicity studies were used to provide more substantial information concerning the suggested relationship between chemicals or mixtures and their known ability to cause tumors in man (Tomatis, 1979). The first test confirming the association between mixtures of the chemicals in coal tars and their carcinogenic effects in man was performed by Yamagiwa and Ichikawa (1915).

Currently, such studies are commonly employed to detect chemicals having carcinogenic activity in animals for the purpose of extrapolation to man (Griesemer and Cueto, 1980).

The appropriateness and use of chronic toxicity/carcinogenicity bio-assays for the purpose of extrapolation has been the subject of several recent articles (Griesemer and Cueto, 1980; Tomatis, 1977a, 1977b, 1979; Tomatis *et al.*, 1978) and will not be dealt with here *per se*. A major concern, when data from a chronic toxicity/carcinogenicity bioassay are used for extrapolation, is whether the animal model is a good predictor of what may occur when humans are exposed to the substance. While definitive evidence to substantiate the carcinogenic effect of a substance in man usually involves epidemiological studies, the results of such studies are also fraught with difficulties (Doll, 1979; NAS, 1979). Tomatis (1979) and Bartsch *et al.* (1982) discussed the correlation between the chemicals or industrial processes that have been associated with the occurrence of cancer in man and the predictive value of laboratory animal studies. Epidemiological studies and/or case reports are available for only about 60 chemicals (of the 532 compounds IARC has evaluated), groups of chemicals, industries or industrial processes; for 22 of these, the available evidence was sufficient to support a causal relationship with the occurrence of cancers in humans. In addition, there is an additional group of five chemicals, groups of chemicals and industries or industrial processes with evidence "almost sufficient" to implicate them as human carcinogens and a group of 13 chemicals for which "suggestive" evidence exists. While there is substantial evidence that arsenic compounds induce skin and lung cancer in man, the available animal studies reviewed by Tomatis (1979) were considered to be negative. A comparison of organ specificities for 15 other chemicals indicated that man and one of the animal species tested have a similarly affected target organ. For the remaining three compounds the authors who conducted the animal studies did not indicate which organs had tumors. While it might be assumed that similar target organs would be affected if the route of exposure was similar, human carcinogens have been found to be carcinogenic when administered to animals via routes other than those by which man is generally exposed. However, it is open to question whether epidemiologists have looked adequately at more than 25% of human carcinogens to determine if they affect more than one tissue. For example, the question of whether the known human bladder carcinogens induce cancer at sites other than the urinary tract has not been adequately addressed. Tomatis *et al.* (1978) noted that multiple target organs occur more frequently in test animals than with man.

It should be noted that experimental evidence for the carcinogenic potential of aflatoxin, 4-aminobiphenyl, bis (chloromethyl) ether, diethylstilbestrol, melphalan, mustard gas, and vinyl chloride preceded evidence for carcinogenic effects in man. However, with some of these chemicals, the first observations of tumor induction in experimental animals did not indicate the target organ subsequently found for man (Tomatis, 1979).

A recent IARC (1982) monograph identifies seven industrial processes and occupational exposures and 23 chemicals and groups of chemicals that are causally associated with cancer in humans. The list does not include known human carcinogens such as tobacco and alcoholic beverages. The monograph identifies 61 chemicals, groups of chemicals, or industrial processes that are probably carcinogenic to humans.

Arnold and Grice (1979) compared interspecies susceptibility of the hamster, mouse and rat to carcinogenic agents and found that the percentage of interspecies predictability ranged from 84 to 90%. Additionally, Purchase (1980) found in his review of carcinogenic compounds that if there was a positive response in one of these species, there was approximately an 85% chance of a positive response in the second species. While some of these species differences are probably attributable to activation or deactivation of the administered material and/or the sensitivity to tissue damage (Reitz *et al.*, 1980), pharmacokinetics, physiological differences and experimental details (Rall, 1977a, 1977b; Tomatis, 1977b), a great deal of research is still required for a better understanding of these differences.

2.18. Overview

Most long-term toxicity/carcinogenicity studies are now designed and conducted according to international guidelines. When studies conform with the principles of GLP (Federal Register, 1978a), their evaluation is greatly facilitated. Conversely, studies that are not designed or conducted in such a fashion are often very difficult to assess and are not appropriate for a final judgment on the chemical's carcinogenic potential in and of themselves.

Properly designed and conducted long-term carcinogenicity experiments may culminate in a wide variety of results. In some instances, the outcome may be clear, as with a carcinogen producing a marked increase in the occurrence of a rare tumor. Other studies, however, may require careful evaluation before a compound can be designated a carcinogen even in the species tested.

The determination of tumor induction in animals ultimately relies upon both biological evaluation and statistical analysis, with the weight of evidence in support of carcinogenicity being greater to the extent that the effects outlined in Section 2.16 are present.

When the results of a chronic carcinogenicity bioassay are to be analyzed, it is important that the original objective of the study be considered. Evidence arising from studies conducted for purposes other than assessing the carcinogenic potential of the test compound *per se* should be considered as ancillary observations that may be useful in attempting to define mechanisms. Such studies include those designed to assess initiation (promotion phenomena) (Cohen *et al.*, 1979b; Hicks *et al.*, 1975), synergism or antagonism (Section V) or reversibility (Arnold *et al.*, 1983).

In some studies, animals with a high spontaneous tumor incidence are observed to have an increased incidence of that lesion in one of the treated groups. The information by itself is of limited use in assessing the carcinogenic potential of the chemical and attempts should be made to determine the likely mechanism of the effect using data from other sources. Whenever there is insufficient evidence of carcinogenicity from a long-term carcinogenicity study, it may be necessary to initiate new and more rigorous studies involving different routes of exposure and dose levels in the same and different strain or species.

A review of all the chemical/biological properties of the test chemical (see Section VII) will aid in an attempt to arrive at the possible mechanism of the effect and will help to define what additional studies may be required.

III. Short-Term Tests

3.1. Introduction

Short-term tests are increasingly used to provide a prescreen for potential carcinogenicity of compounds. Many carcinogens act through the development of a DNA-damaging metabolite (e.g., an 'electrophile'; see Section VI) which binds with cellular macromolecules (Miller and Miller, 1969), the so-called somatic mutation theory (Boveri, 1929). Hence, the detection of genotoxic properties of compounds or their metabolites is one of the important parameters to be investigated.

In the definition of a carcinogen (see Section 6.1), the most important criterion is the biological end result (the development of the tumors), rather than the mechanism of action of the compound giving rise to the tumors. Carcinogens acting through a different "indirect" mechanism, "nongenotoxic" or "epigenetic," come within this definition (Clayson, 1981; Kroes, 1979; Weisburger and Williams, 1978,1980; Williams, 1979a). Thus it is important to emphasize that only genotoxic compounds

will be detected in those short-term tests that are based on the detection of
DNA-damaging or mutagenic properties of chemicals. This is one of the
reasons why carcinogens are not always positive in short-term screening
tests.

3.2. Short-Term Screening Tests

The recognition of metabolic activation in a bacterial mutation system
(Ames *et al.*, 1975) was a major achievement in understanding *in vivo*
systems. Since then, a large number of chemicals have been identified that
could be metabolized *in vitro* to produce positive results in the many
mutagenicity assays subsequently developed.
    Presently available short-term tests measure a variety of end points
including:

• DNA damage and DNA repair;
• mutagenicity;
• chromosome effects;
• transformation of mammalian cells in culture.

Comprehensive reviews of the available assay systems have recently been
published (IARC, 1980b; Williams *et al.*, 1982). Therefore, only some
general remarks will be made here.

3.3. Short-Term Tests to Detect Mutagenicity

These tests can be carried out with prokaryotes (usually bacteria) and
eukaryotes (yeasts, molds, insects or mammalian cells).
    Tests using prokaryotes or eukaryotes are designed to detect different
types of mutations. The special strains of *Salmonella typhimurium* used
in the Ames test have permeable cellular membranes, and strains have
been made repair-deficient to improve the sensitivity of the assays.
Eukaryotes are sometimes preferred since their genetic structure resem-
bles the human genetic structure more than prokaryotes.
    Saccharomyces cerevisiae and *Neurospora crassa* have been the
most commonly used yeast and mold, respectively. Tests to detect
mutagenic activity in mammalian cells are usually carried out with
aneuploid Chinese hamster ovary (CHO) cells (O'Neill *et al.*, 1977), V79
(Chu and Malling, 1968), and L5178 (Clive and Spector, 1975). All the
tests cited previously, using prokaryotes and eukaryotes, are carried out
with and without a metabolic activation system. *Drosophila* offers the
advantage of a P-450 complex type of metabolism in an intact organism.

The prokaryotic assays as well as the eukaryotic yeast mold assays have the advantage of being relatively inexpensive and rapid (2-3 weeks). The *Drosophila* system does not have these advantages, but has the advantage of being able to detect several genetic effects. Mammalian cell systems have the advantage of having a genetic structure similar to man.

3.4. DNA Damage Tests

These tests are especially important since many carcinogens induce damage in cellular DNA when they are metabolized to reactive metabolites (ultimate carcinogens). DNA damage induces unscheduled DNA repair. Therefore, both DNA damage and DNA repair can be measured as parameters in such tests.

Many mammalian cell systems are in use, including human cell cultures. One useful assay is the Williams hepatocyte primary culture/DNA repair test in which the metabolic capability of intact cells is utilized (Williams, 1976, 1977).

3.5. Chromosome Effects

Tests in eukaryotic systems for chromosome effects measure alterations in the structure and number (aneuploidy) of chromosomes and sister chromatid exchange (SCE) (Wolff, 1981). SCE appears to be more sensitive than other chromosome effects. Neither its underlying mechanisms, however, nor those of any of the *in vivo* cytogenetic test systems are understood.

3.6. Cell Transformation Tests

The transformation of mammalian cells in culture is another important parameter in assessing the potential for carcinogenicity. Cell transformation can be detected by morphologic criteria (piling up, criss-cross pattern), growth in soft agar or tumor growth in a syngeneic host or nude (athymic) mice. The cell systems which are presently used are all of non-epithelial nature; whereas, in fact, epithelial cells are to be preferred, especially since most tumors found in man and animals are of epithelial origin.

Most commonly used are the Syrian hamster embryo cell system (Di Paola *et al.*, 1979; Pienta *et al.*, 1977), C_3H 10T½ (Reznikoff *et al.*, 1973), BALB/c 3T3 (Kakunaga, 1973), and BHK_{21}(Dia Mayorca *et al.*, 1973) cell lines.

Some of these systems are variable in their ability to metabolize compounds; therefore, a metabolic activation system should be used. A feature of transformation tests is their potential ability to detect genotoxic and nongenotoxic carcinogens. Cell transformation systems, however, have not been developed to the point where reliable, reproducible results can be obtained in different laboratories; such systems have not been vigorously validated.

3.7. Tests for Tumor Promoters

Several approaches to the detection of promoters have been suggested (Farber and Solt, 1978; Kinsella and Radman, 1978; Murray and Fitzgerald, 1979; Parry *et al.*, 1981; Sivak, 1982; Weinstein *et al.*, 1982; Yotti *et al.*, 1979). Inhibition of cell-cell communication may be an important effect of promoters leading to the escape of initiated cells from restraint by surrounding normal cells (Trosko *et al.*, 1981; Williams, 1981d). In culture systems which measure inhibition of intercellular communication (metabolic cooperation), a variety of tumor promoters have been active (Murray and Fitzgerald, 1979; Trosko *et al.*, 1981; Umeda *et al.*, 1980; Williams *et al.*, 1981; Yotti *et al.*, 1979).

3.8. Predictive Value of Short-Term Screening Tests

Two problems in short-term tests are false positive and false negative results. The performance of short-term tests can be judged by the following criteria (Cooper *et al.*, 1979; de Serres, 1980):

- sensitivity: the proportion of positive results among the recognized carcinogens tested (true positive);
- specificity: the proportion of negative results among the non-carcinogens tested (true negative);
- accuracy: the total proportion of correct results among the total number of carcinogens and noncarcinogens tested. In assessing the predictability of short-term tests, it must be borne in mind that tests for genetic damage can possibly detect only genotoxic carcinogens. Thus, the level of correlation of positive results with carcinogenicity will be a function of the proportion of genotoxins among the carcinogens evaluated.

3.9. Predictive Value of Mutagenicity Tests

Although the *Salmonella*/mammalian microsome assay is the most widely-used system, there is variation in results between laboratories and test protocols (Batzinger *et al.*, 1977). In evaluation of results from several investigators (Bartsch *et al.*, 1980; Brown *et al.*, 1979; Dunkel and Simmon, 1980; Kawachi *et al.*, 1980; McCann *et al.*, 1976; Rinkus and Legator, 1979; Rosenkranz and Poirer, 1979; Simmon, 1979b) it was found that the sensitivity ranges from 61-90%, the specificity from 57-87% and the accuracy from 62-89%. Thus the results of the tests vary considerably. In addition, limited information on other assay systems suggests an error rate of at least this magnitude (Brown *et al.*, 1979; IARC, 1980b; Loprieno, 1980; Rosenkranz and Poirer, 1979; Simmon, 1979a; Vogel *et al.*, 1980).

In the Ames system some compounds are expected to be negative since they are considered to be nongenotoxic (epigenetic) carcinogens, e.g., hormones, anti-hormones, some enzyme-inducing agents, saccharin and nitrilotriacetic acid (NTA). Negative results may also occur because the test is not a perfect predictor. On the other hand, for other compounds such as dimethylhydrazine, the negative results can be explained by the insufficiency of the metabolic system used. In this respect the results of Rinkus and Legator (1979) are of interest. In a study of 465 chemicals in which the carcinogenic activity, chemical structure, and results in the Ames test were compared, there was poor correlation among those chemicals which exhibited less potent carcinogenic activity; many of these compounds are nongenotoxic.

3.10. Predictive Value of DNA Repair Tests

Of the DNA repair systems available, the sensitivity ranges from 62–94% (Martin *et al.*, 1978; Stitch *et al.*, 1976; Swenberg *et al.*, 1979; Williams, 1980a). Williams indicated that some enzyme-inducing compounds such as DDT, DDE and phenobarbital do not induce DNA repair in his system; this again indicates the existence of nongenotoxic carcinogens (Williams, 1979a, 1980b). These tests are also of value in the prediction of possible carcinogenicity (ICPEMC, 1982).

3.11. Predictive Value of Chromosome Tests

It is well-established that chromosome aberrations, aneuploidy and SCE are produced by a variety of carcinogens. Therefore, all have been advocated as end points in carcinogen testing. The production of chromosome aberrations shows a good correlation with carcinogenicity, but the data base is limited (Preston *et al.*, 1981). SCE has been studied more extensively (Wolff and Wiley, 1982) probably because of the greater ease with which SCE's can be measured. In a blind study, Natarajan and Obe (1982) found a 75-80% reliability for both chromosome aberrations and SCE in identifying carcinogens. In the EPA Gene Tox Program (Latt *et al.*, 1981), 40 of 163 compounds evaluated for SCE had available carcinogenesis data. Of these, 25 which were carcinogens produced SCE, while four carcinogens were negative for SCE induction. Three chemicals showed only SCE induction, and seven yielded equivocal results. Thus, while production of chromosome effects is predictive of carcinogenicity, both false positives and false negatives occur.

3.12. Predictive Value of Cell Transformation Tests

Experience with cell transformation systems is limited. Most systems yield satisfactory correlative results only in laboratories where the systems were developed or were in use for a long time.

The Syrian hamster embryo cell system, which has been standardized by Pienta (1980), shows good correlation with carcinogenicity. Certain compounds that were found to be negative in this system were also negative in the mutagenicity and DNA repair systems (hormones and some enzyme-inducing agents). Conversely, other compounds found positive in this system (e.g., diethylstilbestrol, auramine, aminotriazole, ethionine) indicate that the cell transformation system may be able to detect not only genotoxic but also certain nongenotoxic carcinogens. Thus, the potential of such tests in detecting tumor-enhancing properties of chemicals should be investigated. Factors that are not always taken into consideration in the development of appropriate transformation systems include: organ-tissue specificity, species specificity and culture conditions, e.g., medium components, which affect the metabolism and chemical reactions of carcinogens.

3.13. Predictive Value of Tests for Tumor Promoters

The correlation of positive results in systems measuring inhibition of intercellular communication with promoting activity has been good. However, there are few nonphorbol compounds with known promoting action that can be used for validation of this approach.

3.14. Role of Short-Term Tests

Short-term tests have some predictive value in assisting in the detection of potential carcinogens of the genotoxic type. However, no single test has proven adequate for this purpose, and therefore a battery of tests is generally recommended (FSC, 1978; Health Council of the Netherlands, 1980; IARC, 1980b; ICPEMC, 1982; Purchase, 1982; Williams and Weisburger, 1981). Even with the use of a battery, positive results are only an indication of carcinogenic potential.

A second major role for short-term tests is their utility in helping to define carcinogenic mechanisms. Reliable evidence of activity in short-term tests is indicative of genotoxic capability. Such carcinogens presumably operate as initiating agents in tumor induction (Section III) and probably pose a greater risk to humans than do nongenotoxic carcinogens, which operate by indirect mechanisms.

A point to be emphasized, however, is that quantitative results in short-term tests do not necessarily correlate with carcinogenic potency (Purchase, 1982) partly because the system generally used for metabolic activation, the S9 fraction of the rat liver, does not quantitatively metabolize chemicals as do whole cells (Jones *et al.*, 1981; Wright, 1980).

IV. Pharmacokinetics and Metabolism

4.1. Introduction

Pharmacokinetic studies may assist in the interpretation of the results obtained in animal studies, the extrapolation of data to man, and in the validation of mathematical models used in the extrapolation of dose-response data to estimate the risk at low doses. When information is available to indicate that the metabolism and kinetics of a test substance are similar in man and test animals, extrapolation between test species and man is more scientifically defensible. Furthermore, good pharmaco-kinetic data can permit the calculation of a nominal systemic exposure concentration which enables the investigator to obtain comparisons between animals and man on a more rational basis than is possible by using the exposure or dose alone.

However, it should not be assumed that similar kinetic findings in several species guarantees similar biological responses in all species, since these will depend upon the presence at a target site of a given concentration of the test substance or active metabolite and the intrinsic reactivity of the metabolite. The sensitivity of the target sites to respond to a given concentration of the active agent is also a factor which must be considered. For instance, d-amphetamine produces a hyperthermic response in CD_1 mice but not in C_3H mice even though the concentrations of this drug in the brain are comparable in these two strains (Jori and Caccia, 1975). Furthermore, several recent reviews and communications have established that, for a number of chemicals, the kinetic parameters for a given toxicant may differ widely depending on the animal species used in the investigation (Baty, 1979, 1981; Burke and Upshall, 1976; Franklin and Aldridge, 1976; Gillette, 1976; Keck, 1981).

The rates and mechanisms of absorption, distribution, metabolism and excretion are important in understanding the quantitative response of an animal to a given dose, for calculating the effective dose and for extrapolating data obtained in one species to another[1] (Gillette, 1976; NAS, 1980; Withey, 1982). In assessing the effective dose it should be remembered that the dose of the compound administered will undergo metabolism, either to yield a less active or innocuous form (detoxification) or a more potent toxicant (activation). In addition, factors that influence either the mechanism or the rate of absorption, distribution, metabolism and excretion will alter the concentration of active species at reaction sites and hence the magnitude of the response.

4.2. Absorption

There are no general statements that can be made with regard to species differences in absorption. It has been suggested that the rate of uptake of an orally-administered dose in ruminants is slower than in monogastric species due to the dilution factor, a consequence of stomach volume (Keck, 1981). A more important aspect is that some herbivores have active microflora and a pH of about 4 in the stomach, whereas carnivores have no gastric microflora and have a gastric pH of about 1. This means that certain toxicants, especially esters and amides, which undergo microbial hydrolysis and reduction, will be altered in the stomach of ruminant species prior to the absorption of an orally-administered dose. Absorption of the same compounds in carnivores, in the absence of microflora, will be of the unaltered toxicant. A good example is the reduced toxicity of dinitrophenoxy herbicides in ruminants due to their facile reduction to the less potent amino derivatives. The oral LD_{50} for dinitrophenol in the rat, for example, is about 10 mg/kg while the lethal dose for bovines is in excess of 50 mg/kg (Keck, 1981).

---

[1]Unfortunately comparative kinetic analyses in several species including man are available only for very few chemicals showing carcinogenic properties. Therefore, most of the examples in this presentation are taken from various fields of pharmacology and toxicology.

There are other, less precisely understood examples of large inter-species differences in the uptake of orally-administered drugs. The adrenergic blocking agents nadolol and atenolol are completely absorbed from the gastrointestinal tract of the dog, while less than 25% uptake of an orally-administered dose occurs in mice, rats, hamsters, rabbits, rhesus monkeys and man (Dreyfus et al., 1978; Reeves et al., 1978). The anti-inflammatory isoxepac is particularly well-absorbed from the gastro-intestinal tract in dogs, monkeys and man, while uptake is significantly lower in the rat and the rabbit at comparable dose levels (Illing and Fromson, 1978).

4.3. Distribution

Once a toxicant has been absorbed into the systemic circulation, it is distributed to the major organs, tissues and target sites. Species differ-ences with respect to factors affecting distribution can occur as a result of anatomical differences, such as the variation in the ratio of lipid to muscle tissue, or as a result of differences in binding characteristics of the xenobiotic within different physiological compartments. For instance, species like the sheep and the pig have a high fat to muscle ratio and, therefore, require much higher doses of lipid-soluble anesthetic gases than do those with a lower ratio. Within the same species, in particular in man, there is a large variation with respect to the body fat composition, neutral fats constituting some 50% of the body weight of an obese individual as opposed to 20% in a lean person (Klaassen, 1980).

The interaction of xenobiotics with macromolecules (within the physiological compartments to which they are distributed) is also species-dependent. For example, the alkaloid pilocarpine binds to proteins to an increasing extent in the pig, cow, horse, sheep and rabbit. As a direct consequence, species sensitivity to this drug increases in the reverse order (Keck, 1981). Larger doses of ciclazindol are needed to saturate the plasma binding sites in rats compared to monkeys (Swaisband et al., 1977). The affinity of paraquat for human lung tissue is a prominent factor in irreversible pulmonary fibrosis in man, while the lungs of rodents and ruminants do not appear to be affected to any great extent (Smalley and Radelett, 1970).

4.4. Metabolism

The factors which appear to account for the greatest variation between species are the differences in the rate at which a given xenobiotic is metabolized and the presence of different metabolic pathways in the various species. It is important to recognize that metabolism can occur in organs other than the liver, although this organ is regarded as the primary site for most anabolic and catabolic transformations. The formation of Phase I (anabolic) and Phase II (conjugate) metabolites frequently involve reactions with enzymes. Some species may have lower levels of particular enzymes; this will be responsible for a different response to a given dose of a xenobiotic. The drug carbenoxolone, for example, is metabolized quite differently in rats, rabbits and mice, on the one hand, and by dogs, non-human primates and man on the other (Pinder *et al.*, 1976). In addition, species differences in the distribution and excretion rates of metabolites may be as important as in their rates of formation (Caldwell, 1981). Of the various metabolic pathways, those involving the mixed function oxidases and other reactions which involve interaction with tissue oxygen show a marked dependence on species body size and weight (Parke and Ioannides, 1981a; Walker, 1978). Since these reactions play an important role in our present understanding of tumorigenesis, they will be considered later in a separate section.

A wide species variation in enzyme activity is responsible for the 50-fold range in the rate at which hexobarbital is metabolized (Quinn *et al.*, 1958). Phenol is metabolized by different conjugative pathways in different species. The pig and the rat excrete the phenylglucuronide and sulfate as the principal metabolites, but the rate of excretion in sheep is some 12% faster due to the formation of the phenylphosphate metabolite not found in the former species (Kao *et al.*, 1979). The rat lacks the ability to N-hydroxylate aliphatic amines; the guinea pig cannot N-hydroxylate aromatic amides nor can it produce mercapturic acids. Cats are unable to form the glucuronide of phenols or aromatic acids. The dog cannot acetylate primary amino groups effectively nor can it effect some kinds of acyclic hydroxylation.

An important difference between small rodents and higher mammals is that the former tend to use glutathione rather than water for detoxification; the ratio of glutathione transferase to epoxide hydrase activities is much higher in the rat and mouse than in non-human primates and man. It should be noted that the depletion of intracellular glutathione produces marked metabolic and structural changes in the cell which makes it more vulnerable to the action of oxidants and free radicals. The rat and mouse thereby use valuable protective materials as their first line of defense, while man and primates use glutathione only as a reserve after epoxide hydrase and water have exercised the primary protective effect (Pacifici *et al.*, 1981).

Attempts to mimic the pharmacokinetic and metabolic patterns in man by using non-human primates have not always met with success.

Striking differences between monkeys and man have been found in the metabolism of meperidine (Caldwell et al., 1979). An evaluation of various species as possible metabolic surrogates for man has been summarized by Smith and Caldwell (1976). For the 23 compounds cited, the best metabolic model for the human was the monkey on 17 occasions. By contrast the rat provided a good model for only four compounds and was invalid for eight others. Other non-primate species provided suitable metabolic models on only five occasions and were inappropriate for six compounds.

It has been suggested that a general approach to minimize species differences with man should take into account all of the pharmacokinetic mechanisms involved (Gillette, 1976, 1977). Gillette points out that in cases where the duration of activity of a xenobiotic is proportional to its elimination rate, as it is in the case of hexobarbitone (Quinn et al., 1958), the pharmacologic activity is due to the intrinsic activity of the drug itself. In any event it is possible to minimize the species differences by varying either the dose or the dose interval. This may allow the same steady state levels to be achieved in any species. In the case where particular metabolic pathways are available in one species but not in another, Gillette suggests that similar effects might be achieved in both species by the co-administration of metabolites, together with the test compound, in the metabolically-deficient species.

Gillette has also discussed the specific cases of liver necrosis caused by paracetamol (Mitchell et al., 1973; Potter et al., 1974), the carcinogenic action of 2-acetylaminofluorene (2-AAF) (Miller, 1970) and liver necrosis induced by halogenated aromatic hydrocarbons (Brodie et al., 1971) as examples where mechanisms of action are known. In the case of the carcinogenic action of 2-AAF, a series of consecutive and simultaneous reactions occur in six stages. The necessary equations to allow a calculation of the ultimate effective fraction of the administered dose are given. In some respects this approach can be simplified; useful information about saturation of metabolic pathways and a rationale for changes in the slope of dose-response curves are given by Gehring et al. (1979) and Ramsey and Reitz (1981).

4.5. Mixed Function Oxidases

The microsomal monoxygenase systems, or mixed function oxidases, are known to play a very important part both in the activation and in the detoxification of pre-carcinogens and carcinogens (Parke, 1981a; Parke and Ioannides, 1981a). Empirically developed relationships are customarily employed to relate dose and effect; the dose can be expressed as the amount administered either per unit body weight or per unit of body surface area (Federal Register, 1978b). While many toxicity parameters and biological constants of mammals correlate quite well, some 15-20% of substances fail to conform to a linear relationship with either expression of linear dosage (Filov et al., 1979; Krasovskii, 1976).

Experimental observations (Parke and Ioannides, 1981a; Walker, 1978) show that the metabolism of xenobiotic chemicals by the mixed function oxidases occurs more rapidly in smaller species, such as the mouse, and proceeds more slowly with increasing body weight. As a consequence, environmental chemicals which are activated to proximate and ultimate carcinogens by the mixed function oxidases are more readily activated by small mammals, like the mouse and rat, than by larger species like man, non-human primates and dogs. Conversely, chemicals which are detoxified by the mixed function oxidases are altered more readily in smaller animals. The reason for the proportionality of the activity of mixed function oxidases to body weight is probably that it is dependent on other factors besides the concentration of tissue oxygen. The smaller the body weight of the animal species, the greater the oxygen tension is as a consequence of various physiological factors (Booth et al., 1967).

Toxicity of oxygen in the tissues is another factor related to mixed function oxidase activity which should be considered. The free radical theory of oxygen toxicity attributes the damaging effects of hyperoxia to the production of reactive species like the singlet oxygen, hydroxyl radical and superoxide anion. These reactive species can inactivate enzymes in the cell, damage DNA and disorganize intracellular metabolism and regulation (Frank and Massaro, 1980). They may be generated by the action of flavoproteins, or by the action of hemes, or simply by the presence of inorganic iron or other heavy metals.

The usual life span of particular animal species also depends on tissue oxygen tension and thus on body weight (Schwartz and Moore, 1977, 1979). Accordingly, the smaller the species is, the higher the tissue oxygen tension, the greater the extent of formation of active oxygen species, the greater the oxygen toxicity, and the shorter the life span. If current theories are correct which relate to those chemical carcinogens requiring intermediate formation of oxygen radicals, then not only will chemical carcinogens be more readily activated in small species but active oxygen species will also be generated with greater facility in the smaller animals (Stier et al., 1980). One might, therefore, speculate that the carcinogenic potency of xenobiotics requiring the interaction of active oxygen species should be much greater in small mammals, like the mouse and the rat, than in larger species, such as primates and man. In addition, the concentration of the terminal microsomal oxygenase cytochrome

P-450 has also been shown to be dependent on tissue oxygen tension; therefore, smaller animals may have a higher P-450 tissue concentration and a higher rate of oxidative metabolism for activation or detoxification (Langmuir et al., 1980).

Numerous pre-carcinogens are known to require activation to the ultimate carcinogen by the mixed function oxidases of the liver cell endoplasmic reticulum (Ioannides and Parke, 1980), although the dialkylnitrosamines may be activated by cytosolic or mitochondrial enzymes (Magee et al., 1976). The activities of the microsomal mixed function oxidases depend on the genetics of the species, as well as on age, sex, nutritional status and environment. There is good evidence that the activities of the various microsomal cytochromes and other oxidases which govern detoxification/activation reactions are determined partly by genetics and partly by environmental experience. On exposure to polycyclic aromatic hydrocarbons particularly, changes occur to cause the conversion of hepatic cytochrome P-450 activity to that of cytochrome P-448, a process which might be considered to be autocatalytic since cytochrome P-448 appears to be involved more in the activation of carcinogens than in their detoxification (Levin et al., 1977; Parke and Ioannides, 1981a). The composition of membranes of the endoplasmic reticulum, particularly the lipid components, may also greatly affect the activity of the mixed function oxidases.

An essential constituent of hepatic endoplasmic reticulum is the phospholipid and phosphatidylcholine content. When phosphatidylcholine is replaced by phosphatidylethanolamine, decoupling of the cytochrome P-450 from its flavoprotein reductase occurs, with accompanying changes in the nature and extent of enzymic mixed function oxidation (Parke, 1981b). Sex differences with respect to mixed function oxidase activity occur in the rat and other species. This has also been attributed to differences in the lipid composition of the endoplasmic reticulum, and possibly to the replacement of phosphatidylcholine by phosphatidylethanolamine, because of an inherent defect in the ability of the rat to synthesize choline (Pani et al., 1978). It has also been suggested that a progressive replacement of phosphatidylcholine by phosphatidylethanolamine occurs during the aging process in rats and other mammals, and that this may have similar effects on the extent and mode (detoxification or activation) of mixed function oxidase activity (Parke, 1981b).

The microsomal monooxygenase systems have also attracted considerable attention as a consequence of interactions that induce or antagonize their activity (Gelboin, 1976; Remmer, 1969; Testa and Jenner, 1976). Almost any lipid substance will cause some degree of induction, and xenobiotics like the organochlorine pesticides, which are slowly eliminated from the body, have a larger capacity for induction than others which are rapidly excreted. More specific microsomal enzymes are induced by the polycyclic aromatic hydrocarbons than are induced by drugs such as phenobarbital and amphetamines, but no structure-activity relationships have been clearly established. Most studies have involved the microsomal oxidases of the liver, although extra-hepatic monoxygenase systems have been defined for lung, skin and intestine; these may be quite different from those of the liver (Alvares, 1977; Grafstrom et al., 1977; Wallenberg and Ullrich, 1977).

A number of factors can alter the extent of induction. Usually long exposure is required for an agent to induce hepatic response (Remmer, 1969), although 3-methylcholanthrene exerts its maximum effect within 24 hours after exposure. The maximum effect of chlordane is evident only after several weeks of exposure (Testa and Jenner, 1976). A number of well-known mixed function oxidase inducers, like SKF-525A (diethylaminoethyl-2,2-diphenylvalerate hydrochloride), and 1,3 benzodioxoles, are biphasic in their action; they cause inhibition during the first 12 hours post-administration, followed by a marked stimulation (Wilkinson, 1976).

4.6. Covalent Binding

Some carcinogens, such as epoxides, β-lactones and methane sulfonate esters, are believed to exert their effect by direct covalent binding with intracellular proteins or DNA or by forming ligand complexes with cytochrome P-450. Some chemicals can form free radicals, which are less discriminating than are electrophiles in reacting with centers on macromolecules.

It is now believed that enzymes which cause the detoxification of chemicals are only rarely the same enzymes which cause activation. Evidence is accumulating that cytochrome P-450 is generally involved in detoxification reactions, whereas activation is usually caused by cytochrome P-448 (Parke and Ioannides, 1981a). Since there are pronounced species differences in the predominance of these enzymes (both microsomal and cytosolic), major differences in the ratio of detoxification/activation of pre-carcinogens may occur in different species. For example, the mouse has a preponderance of high-spin cytochrome P-450 in the liver which readily activates carcinogenic polycyclic hydrocarbons. Unlike the situation in the rat, cytochrome P-450 in the mouse is not activated by prior administration of 3-methylcholanthrene or Aroclor.

4.7. Excretion

Both rates and mechanisms of excretion can vary among species. Water soluble xenobiotics and metabolites are excreted largely via the kidney. Renal tubular reabsorption is a well-established phenomenon which can be an active and saturable transport process, and, therefore, liable to saturation in the presence of high xenobiotic concentrations (Jusko and Levy, 1970). Weak acids, like barbiturates, salicylates, aryloxyacid herbicides and coumarin anticoagulants are reabsorbed to a much greater extent in carnivorous species, since these animals have a relatively low urinary pH which favors the un-ionized form; it is the un-ionized form which is reabsorbed (Keck, 1981).

Biliary excretion is an important route. Examples of species differences due to alternative biliary excretion mechanisms abound, and the reasons for this are still largely unknown (Smith, 1973). Biliary excretion occurs in the rat and dog to a much greater extent than in the rabbit, monkey or man. There appears to be a reasonably well-defined biliary excretion threshold of approximately 300 molecular weight for the rat and dog and around 450 for the rabbit, monkey and man.

There are a number of examples where biliary excretion plays an important role in determining the elimination kinetics and toxicity (Baty, 1979, 1981). The drug hycanthone is eliminated almost entirely via the bile in dogs and rabbits, while in cats and monkeys only urinary excretion is observed. This could account for the high toxicity of hycanthone in cats and monkeys (Davison *et al.*, 1977). Substances that are metabolized to a great extent, like the dyestuff Rose Bengal, may be excreted exclusively via the bile at widely differing rates. In the case of Rose Bengal, the half lives for its excretion in the guinea pig, rat, rabbit and dog are 17, 30, 30 and 46 minutes, respectively. Since biliary excretion is the major route for some species, while it plays a minor role in others, large excretion rate differences occur. For example, the substances ouabain, procaine and bromosulfone phthalein are excreted much faster by the rat than by the dog; less than 3% of an administered dose is excreted by the dog via the bile (Klaassen, 1980).

Special considerations are necessary for two pharmacokinetic mechanisms. The first is a consequence of the inter-species variability in the biliary excretion of xenobiotics, as well as their metabolites and conjugates into the lower gastrointestinal tract. Bacterial-assisted degradation of glucuronides and other conjugates permits the reabsorption of many active compounds into the systemic circulation via the portal vein. Thus the reabsorption of some compounds results in a greater persistence within the system. Such is the case with the antibiotic chloramphenicol which is liberated from its glucuronide conjugate and reabsorbed (Glazko *et al.*, 1952).

The other mechanism is known as the "first pass effect" (Baty, 1979, 1981). It is primarily involved with those xenobiotics which are extensively metabolized by the liver. This effect occurs when a compound is absorbed from the gastrointestinal tract, taken up into the portal system, passed through the liver, and metabolized. This is in contrast to pulmonary or intravenous administration where the entire dose is carried and divided, more or less equally after venous uptake, to the major organs by the systemic circulation. A good example of the importance of this effect is seen with the potent analgesic meptazinol (Franklin and Aldridge, 1976). The administration of a 25 mg/kg oral dose to rats and monkeys gave peak plasma levels which were 17 times higher in the rat than in the monkey, due to a large first pass effect in the latter species.

V. Synergism and Antagonism

5.1. Introduction

With thousands of natural and synthetic chemicals in use, it is likely that some humans will be exposed to two or more potentially injurious chemicals simultaneously or closely in time. Relevant to this, and of direct concern to the research toxicologist, is the potential for synergism or antagonism when the experimental animal is inadvertently exposed to one or more chemicals other than the test material, or when the experimental design includes exposure to more than one foreign compound. A similar problem arises for a toxicologist in attempting risk assessment and extrapolation of experimental animal data to man for a particular chemical, when man, in everyday activities and through varying lifestyles, is exposed to a multitude of chemicals in an ever changing array of doses and frequencies.

Toxicological interactions are those situations in which exposure to two or more chemicals results in a qualitatively or quantitatively altered biological response relative to that predictable from the actions of each single chemical. Such multiple chemical exposures may be simultaneous or sequential, and the altered response may be greater (synergistic) or smaller (antagonistic) than that predicted from the properties of the individual substances.

5.2. Synergism

When two compounds are given simultaneously or sequentially, and the effect is greater than would be expected from the potency of the individual compounds, this is referred to as synergism.

The majority of synergistic interactions appears to involve the inhibition of xenobiotic-metabolizing enzymes. Two of the best-known examples in toxicology involve insecticides: methylene-dioxyphenol synergists and the potentiation of the insecticide malathion by a large number of other organophosphate compounds. Synergistic action is often seen with drugs. Almost all cases in which hexobarbital sleeping time or zoxazolamine paralysis time have been increased by other chemicals could be described as synergism due to a blockade of liver microsomal enzymes by the interacting chemical. Synergism may result from competition for binding sites on plasma proteins or from competition for an active secretion mechanism in the renal tubule. The increased incidence of lung cancer resulting from occupational exposure to asbestos in smokers is an example of synergistic effects in the workplace. Synergism may also occur when a given chemical enhances tissue microsomal enzymes (induction) if the interacting chemical requires metabolic activation to bring about its pharmacological or toxic effects.

5.3. Antagonism

Antagonism is the condition in which the toxicity of two or more compounds administered together or sequentially is less than would be expected from a consideration of their toxicities when administered individually. This includes cases where one chemical may prevent the absorption of another chemical, either decreasing the intestinal transit time (e.g., antagonism resulting from the combined use of laxatives and steroidal contraceptive drugs) or by competing with a transport mechanism (e.g., DOPA and α-methyl dopa).

Reduced absorption can occur when two chemicals are injected together subcutaneously. For example, calcium reduces the entry of reserpine into the circulation resulting in a reduced pharmacological effect of reserpine (Manara et al., 1976). Lowered toxicity can also result from induction of detoxifying enzymes. The reduction of hexobarbital sleeping time and the reduction of zoxazolamine paralysis time by prior treatment with phenobarbital are obvious examples of such induction effects at the level of pharmacologic action. Protection from the carcinogenic actions of benzo(a)pyrene, aflatoxin, and diethylnitrosamine by phenobarbital are examples at the level of chronic toxicity (Hodgson, 1980).

In some cases, the mechanism involved may be more complex. For instance, phenobarbital antagonizes the anti-tumor and the immuno-depressant effect of cyclophosphamide. Phenobarbital increases the formation of the alkylating metabolites responsible for the toxic effects of cyclophosphamide and enhances the metabolism of these alkylating agents (Garattini et al., 1975).

Antagonism may also result from inhibition of metabolism of a drug which requires biotransformation to exhibit its effect. For example, the covalent binding of benzo(a)pyrene to DNA is antagonized by clotri-mazole, an inhibitor of mixed function monoxygenases (Kahl et al., 1980).

In other cases, the duration of action characterizes the antagonism. A short-acting drug may antagonize the action of a long-acting drug with a similar effect. Pertinent examples in this respect are the antagonism between tetrabenazine and reserpine, two releasers of monoamines (Manara and Garattini, 1967) and tranylcypromine and iproniazide, two monoamineoxidase inhibitors (Pletscher and Besendorf, 1959). These effects are probably due to the temporary occupation of active sites by one drug during the period in which the second drug is metabolized to inactive compounds. Salicylate inhibits the platelet anti-aggregating effect of aspirin in vitro and in vivo by occupying the active sites of cyclo-oxygenase, a key enzyme for the formation of thromboxane ($TxBA_2$), which is a powerful endogenous aggregating agent for platelets (Dejana et al., 1982).

Several different types of antagonism important in toxicology do not involve xenobiotic metabolism. These include competition for receptor sites, such as the competition between CO and O_2 in CO poisoning, and conditions in which one toxicant combines non-enzymatically with another to reduce its toxic effects, such as in the chelation of metal ions. Physiological antagonism is the result of two agonists acting on the same physiological system but producing opposite effects.

5.4. Predicting Interactions

Three basic principles are important in considering the joint toxic action of chemicals (Gillette and Mitchell, 1975; Schand et al., 1975): relative affinities of the individual chemicals for sites of action; relative affinities for sites of loss; and intrinsic activity of the chemicals at their sites of action. Since there are a limited number of sites of action or of loss within any organism, there is a limiting dosage range within which synergism or antagonism can be demonstrated. Interactions can result from the quantity of an active form of one or more chemicals available to a pool of critical cellular macromolecules being altered by one or more other chemicals. Alternatively, the reactivity of critical macromolecules with the active form(s) of exogenous chemicals can be altered by one or more other chemicals each of which may or may not be capable of eliciting a response.

At least three general mechanisms of reactions among chemicals are involved in interactions (Murphy, 1980):

Chemical reactions. One chemical may react directly with another such that potentially injurious forms never reach macromolecular reaction sites within cells. Neutralization reactions among acids and bases and chelation reactions with heavy metals are examples. Antagonism may also occur when a chemical is adsorbed to another material. For instance, charcoal antagonizes the toxicity of 2,3,7,8-tetrachlorodibenzo-p-dioxin (TCDD) (Manara *et al.*, 1982) and cholestyramine reduces the toxic effects of kepone (Boylan *et al.*, 1978).

Chemical competition at macromolecules. There may be varying relative affinities of exogenous chemicals for a limited number of reaction sites to macromolecules. Competition for binding or reaction at various sites may result in enhanced or reduced toxicity; knowing the nature of the chemicals and their reaction kinetics at these sites allow for the possibility of predicting toxicological consequences.

Altered cellular reactivity or responsiveness. Cells and tissues may be affected by one chemical so that the response of the tissue to a second chemical is altered. Initiation and promotion of carcinogenesis, induction of biotransformation enzymes, and alterations in the repair of a cellular lesion are examples of general mechanisms.

The mechanisms involved in synergism or antagonism are often very complex; the specific chemical or biological information required to define these mechanisms is not always available. When mechanisms for particular chemicals are defined, extrapolation from animals to man becomes feasible. Other chemicals to which man is exposed might well influence the defined effects.

An important goal for toxicologists is the development of an adequate pharmacologic data base for chemicals which will permit reasonable estimates of the potential for interaction.

5.5. Testing of Mixtures

Complex mixtures of chemicals present very difficult toxicity and carcinogenicity testing problems. Chemicals in such mixtures may interact *in vivo* to enhance or inhibit response in the test animal or system. Hence quantitative and qualitative differences in the composition of mixtures would be expected to affect test results.

The expert panel for the U.S. EPA "Workshop on Short-Term Bioassays for Estimating Carcinogenic Risk" (1982) noted that the large-scale testing of complex mixtures of variable composition (air, drinking water, or sewage treatment plant effluent) has proven to be impractical. The panel recommended that the matrix approach for estimating carcinogenic risk of mixtures, at its present state of development, should not be used as a risk assessment tool.

VI. Mechanisms of Action

6.1. Definition of a Carcinogen

Several definitions have been used for chemical carcinogens. Some authorities believe that only malignant tumors should be used to define a carcinogen (Clayson, 1962; Health Council of the Netherlands, 1980; Kroes, 1979). Others would include the production of both benign and malignant tumors (Health and Welfare Canada, 1975; Weisburger and Williams, 1980), especially if these tumors arise from a common cell type, while still others believe that benign tumors by themselves are adequate. Vesselinovitch's work with the mouse liver appears to show that hepatocellular hyperplasia, adenoma and carcinoma represent three distinct morphologic and biologic entities. This suggests that only a fraction of the early lesions in the mouse liver are precursors of hepatocellular carcinoma (Vesselinovitch, 1983). IARC (1972) notes that common usage of the term "carcinogen" has led to its use in denoting induction of various types of neoplasms.

These various definitions are not mutually exclusive, since certain types of benign tumors may progress to malignancy. However, if only benign tumors are induced, additional studies are required before the chemical is labelled a carcinogen. Although benign tumors lack the capacity of malignant tumors to invade normal tissues and/or metastasize, they can be a detriment to health and result in death of the host. Therefore, in this document both benign and malignant tumors arising from the same cell type and representing a spectrum of change may be considered as indicators of carcinogenicity.

A carcinogen is an agent that increases the rate of cancer formation in a tissue. The increased rate of tumor formation may be recognized by:

- the development of neoplasms not seen in untreated animals;
- a statistically significant increase in the number of treated animals with tumors of a type occurring in controls;
- induction of rare malignant tumor types;
- evidence of a dose-response relationship;
- a statistically significant increase in the within-organ multiplicity of a tumor type over that seen in controls;
- a decrease in the latency of tumor development from that observed in untreated animals;
- a shift from benign to malignant tumors arising from a given cell type;
- combinations of the above criteria (see also Section 2.16).

While each of these may be used in the interpretation of carcinogenicity, a general increase in tumor incidence without a significant increase in the incidence of any one type of tumor would require further investigation before it could be used to suggest that a chemical is carcinogenic.

6.2. Mechanisms of Action

In recent years a body of opinion has developed that suggests a variety of mechanisms by which carcinogens may exert their effects (Clayson, 1981; Health Council of the Netherlands, 1978; Pitot and Sirica, 1980; Weisburger and Williams, 1980). If this is true, the different mechanisms need to be defined in order to determine whether there should be different approaches to risk estimation for human exposure to carcinogens. It is apparent that a threshold can be demonstrated for certain agents which operate through indirect mechanisms. Because of this, a dose level that would not be expected to induce cancer can be defined. The resolution of this problem is of great importance to carcinogen regulation, because it may help to distinguish those animal carcinogens that do pose a serious risk to the human population from those which do not.

Unfortunately, present knowledge of carcinogenic mechanisms is still fragmentary. It is, therefore, necessary to base methods for the classification of carcinogens on broadly-based concepts rather than on a detailed knowledge of the mechanisms of carcinogenesis. There are two such concepts that have received attention:

- the two-stage model proposed for mouse skin by Berenblum and Shubik (1947a, 1947b, 1949) and subsequently shown to be valid for several other tissues (Clifton and Sridharin, 1975; Hicks et al., 1978;

Peraino *et al.*, 1975; Reddy *et al.*, 1978; Witschi and Lock, 1978);

• the biochemical approach originating in the work of the Millers (Miller and Miller, 1976). This stresses the relevance of metabolic activation of pro-carcinogens, interaction with DNA, DNA damage, and translation of the damage by DNA replication. The proposed result of this is genetically altered cells, among which are believed to be the cells that lead to frank neoplasia.

In combining these two approaches to carcinogenesis it may be suggested that the first stage of carcinogenesis, called initiation by Berenblum and Shubik (1947a, 1947b), consists of metabolic activation of the pro-carcinogen, DNA interaction and fixation of the effect. The second stage of carcinogenesis, promotion, represents the outgrowth of the initiated cells.

There is considerable current interest concerning oncogenes and the role these play in the causation of cancer. Oncogenes are discrete segments of DNA which can transform some kinds of normal cells into malignant neoplastic cells (Astrin and Rothberg, 1983; Reddy *et al.*, 1982a; Shih and Weinberg, 1982; Tabin *et al.*, 1982). The means by which an oncogene causes the phenotypic characteristics of cancer cells is unknown.

A number of normal cellular genes have now been shown to possess oncogenic potential when abnormally expressed. These genes have been identified by homology to the transforming genes of certain retroviruses (Astrin and Rothberg, 1983; Eva, 1982; Marx, 1982; Sheiness and Bishop, 1979; Spector *et al.*, 1978; Stehelin *et al.*, 1976). Their biological activity has been demonstrated by the ability of isolated tumor DNA to transform certain cultured cells such as NIH 3T3 or LtK- mouse cells; this process is termed transfection (Blair *et al.*, 1981; Cooper, 1981; Krontiris and Cooper, 1981; Shih *et al.*, 1979). Thus carcinogenesis, whether "spontaneous," or induced by viruses or chemicals, appears to involve dominant genetic alterations which result in activation of cellular transforming genes. The mechanism by which chemicals activate these genes is probably a function of their genotoxic properties and involves either mutations or minor gene rearrangements rather than gene amplification (Reddy *et al.*, 1982a; Tabin *et al.*, 1982). The long latent period of neoplasia and the phenomenon of tumor promotion further suggest that the sequential activation of a number of different oncogenes may also occur. It is, therefore, evident that the batteries of short-term tests as presently formulated are likely suitable to identify compounds capable of activating these transforming oncogenes.

6.3. Genotoxic and Nongenotoxic (Epigenetic) Carcinogens

The concept that the initiation phase of cancer induction involves DNA interaction of the carcinogen, and possibly the fixation of the damage as a mutation, provides an explanation for the success of genetic damage tests in identifying carcinogens (de Serres and Ashby, 1981b; IARC, 1980b; San and Stich, 1982; Williams, 1980c). Some carcinogens, however, do not induce positive responses in short-term tests. Proposals have been made to categorize carcinogens as genotoxic or nongenotoxic (epigenetic) on the basis of their capacity to damage DNA (Kroes, 1983; Weisburger and Williams, 1980).

Several authors have outlined reasons for considering DNA a critical target of some carcinogens:

- many carcinogens are also mutagens;
- defects in DNA repair (such as that seen in xeroderma pigmentosum) predispose to cancer development;
- several heritable or chromosomal abnormalities predispose to cancer development;
- initiated (dormant) tumor cells are persistent (which is most easily explained by a change in DNA);
- most, if not all, cancers display chromosomal abnormalities;
- many cancers display aberrant gene expression.

Agents which express genotoxic properties generally share several common characteristics:

- they are either electrophilic molecules, or they are capable of metabolic conversion to electrophilic molecules or free radicals, or they may initiate formation of endogenous free radicals (Miller, 1978);
- DNA isolated from cells of animals exposed to these agents can often be shown to be altered, either by the demonstration of covalent adducts of the carcinogen with nucleic acid bases (FSC, 1978; Lutz, 1979; Pegg and Hui, 1978), or by the demonstration of changes in physical stability of the DNA (i.e., breakdown of the DNA to smaller molecular weight entities upon isolation (Zubroff and Sarma, 1976);
- they often induce measurable unscheduled DNA synthesis (DNA repair synthesis), either in primary hepatocyte cultures or in whole animals (Arfellini *et al.*, 1978; Reitz *et al.*, 1980b; Stich and Klesser, 1974);
- they are capable of inducing mutations in prokaryotic and eukaryotic cell test systems such as *Salmonella typhimurium, Escherichia coli,* Chinese hamster ovary cells, or *Drosophila melanogaster*;

- many of these agents cause chromosomal abnormalities;
- many of these agents induce malignant transformation, although this may also be induced by some nongenotoxic chemicals.

The observation that a chemical has several of the properties on this list suggests a genotoxic mode of action. In addition to the formation of adducts to DNA by the agent or its active metabolites, other biochemical mechanisms for genotoxicity have been suggested, e.g., the activation of tissue oxygen (Frank and Massaro, 1980; Trotter, 1980), the formation of stabilized spin-trap radicals from active metabolites of the genotoxic chemical (Stier, 1980), and the initiation of radical-generating mechanisms by flavoprotein reduction of quinones and quinonimine metabolites (Tunek et al., 1980). If tissue oxygen is involved in the mechanism, genotoxic effects should be most evident in smaller animals, such as in mice, because tissue oxygen concentration varies inversely with body weight (Booth et al., 1967).

Genotoxic carcinogens usually, but not always, belong to certain structural classes such as polycyclic aromatic hydrocarbons, aromatic amines, N-nitroso compounds or aflatoxins. Because these structures, to some extent, define the mechanism by which the agents are metabolically activated (this being the major distinction between them) chemical structure may be an appropriate preliminary basis for classification of genotoxic chemicals.

In addition to genotoxic mechanisms, it is clear that effects other than direct alteration of DNA can modify the tumorigenic process. For example, Berenblum (1929) reported the induction of tumors after repeated freezing of mouse skin with solid carbon dioxide where no chemical treatment was involved. Apparent lack of genotoxicity may mask an indirect effect, such as aberrant methylation (Barrows and Shank, 1981). Agents that do not damage DNA directly or through metabolites may alter the fidelity of DNA replication. This is the case with mutagenic/carcinogenic metals that have been shown to affect the fidelity of DNA synthesis in vitro (Loeb et al., 1981; Sirover and Loeb, 1976). Phenomena that have collectively been considered to involve "non-genotoxic" or "epigenetic" processes (Weisburger and Williams, 1980) may be involved in enhancing the spontaneous rates of tumor formation in a bioassay (Health Council of the Netherlands, 1980). Nongenotoxic carcinogens are characterized by a variety of biological properties that are believed to underlie their tumorigenicity. Several examples of critical biological activity are as follows:

- stimulation of cellular proliferation by cytotoxicity and regeneration following chemical treatment (Berenblum, 1944), partial hepatec-

tomy (Craddock and Frei, 1974), or physical or chemical trauma;
- "promotion", e.g., phorbol derivatives (Boutwell, 1974; Diamond *et al.*, 1978, 1980; Sivak, 1982) and indole alkaloids (Fisher *et al.*, 1982); stress (Riley, 1981; Sklar and Anisman, 1981; Visintainer *et al.*, 1982) (for detailed consideration see Section 2.13);
- immune status, e.g., by corticosteroids, aging or stress (Riley, 1981) (for detailed consideration see Section 2.13);
- hormonal balance, e.g., diethylstilbestrol, antithyroid substances, (IARC, 1974a, 1979b) and thyroid status (Vonderhaar and Greco, 1982); prolactin (Welsch and Nagasawa, 1977) (for detailed consideration see Section 2.13);
- nutritional factors, including deficiencies (Parke and Ioannides, 1981b) and hyperalimentation (Tannenbaum and Silverstone, 1957);
- physical irritation, e.g., bladder stones, subcutaneous sarcoma from macromolecular compounds (Boorman and Hollander, 1974; Clayson, 1979; Melnick *et al*, 1984; National Toxicology Program, 1983; Ott, 1970; Thomas *et al.*, 1977);
- enzyme modification, e.g., phenobarbitone and Aroclor.

Pathological effects observed in animal bioassays may indicate that one or more of these factors is likely to be involved. In other cases, detailed qualitative or quantitative information on the acute or chronic biochemical, physiological or morphological effects of the agent may have to be obtained to determine the probable mechanism of action of nongenotoxic carcinogens (Clayson, 1981; Gehring and Blau, 1977; Health Council of the Netherlands, 1980; Kroes, 1979; Weisburger and Williams, 1980). Thus subclassification of chemicals as nongenotoxic carcinogens should include a detailed consideration of their biological effects.

Important information concerning the mechanism of action of a chemical may be obtained in a properly conducted two-stage bioassay. Materials which increase tumor incidence with prolonged administration, only following administration of a genotoxic agent, and not when administered before the genotoxic agent, are characterized as "promoters" and may or may not be genotoxic in and of themselves. Agents which can prepare or "initiate" animals for tumor development in an otherwise nontumorigenic regimen (e.g., multiple applications of 12-0-tetradecanoyl phorbal-13-acetate (TPA)) very well have significant genotoxic activity. However, it must not be overlooked that genotoxic agents themselves may stimulate carcinogenesis resulting from limited application of another genotoxic carcinogen. Therefore, it is essential to verify the lack of genotoxicity of agents which appear to act as promoters.

6.4. Testing for Genotoxic Carcinogens

Tests for genotoxicity contain two components: the organisms in which the genetic changes are expressed, and a system that is capable of converting the pro-genotoxic agent into its active electrophilic or free radical form. Over 100 tests systems have been proposed in the scientific literature (Hollstein *et al.*, 1979). The two components in the test system may each vary considerably in their complexity: the mutable organism may be prokaryotic, eukaryotic unicellular, or eukaryotic multicellular. The metabolizing system may be a subcellular preparation, whole cells, tissue slices or intact tissues in living animals. Genetic end points are likewise varied, including: point mutations, deletions, additions, chromosome breaks or transpositions, SCE, other chromosome aberrations, formation of micronuclei, cell transformation and induction of DNA repair synthesis. With our present experience of these tests, some nongenotoxic carcinogens may be expected to give a minimum of positive genotoxicity results; criteria need to be established to assess the significance of these data (Upton *et al.*, 1984).

6.5. Testing for Nongenotoxic Carcinogens

If a nongenotoxic mechanism is suspected, attempts should be made to ascertain if one of the factors outlined under 6.3 is involved (e.g., physical irritation, stress, hormonal imbalance). An appraisal of the chemical and biological data may provide clues as to possible mechanisms or indicate the nature of additional studies required to define the mechanism.

Attempts to define the mechanism involve determination of the sequence of pathological events that culminates in the formation of a neoplasm. For example, it may be determined that a chemical causes continuous irritation or excessive levels of hormone production leading to hyperplasia of stroma or parenchyma. If the stimulation is sustained, then at some point reversibility may be lost, resulting in what could properly be called "neoplasia."

The nature of the conversion from a hyperplastic cell to a benign or malignant cell is not well understood. However, if a threshold can be defined for the hyperplastic response then a no-effect level can be determined and an appropriate safety factor to permit the use of the chemical can be applied.

Animal tests provide a means for defining nongenotoxic carcinogens. The initiation/promotion model introduced by Berenblum and Shubik (1947a, 1947b, 1949) may be appropriate, but a conventional chronic bioassay may also indicate promotional activity. In the initiation/ promotion bioassay the animals are first exposed to a limited, marginally-tumorigenic dose of a genotoxic carcinogen, followed by exposure to the test agent. The object of this is to demonstrate whether or not the second treatment enhances tumorigenesis. If the test is positive, the test agent may possess promotional activity. In a normal bioassay, initiation may have occurred accidentally (Boutwell, 1974; Roe et al., 1979), or the agent may enhance the development of "spontaneous" tumor occurrence (Clayson, 1981; Clayson et al., 1983).

Short-term tests are presently being developed for the detection of agents capable of promoting carcinogenesis (Sivak, 1982). These tests still require validation. They are dependent on the demonstration of a critical property common to most promoting agents that may be detected in vitro such as cell-to-cell communication.

6.6. Implications of Genotoxic and Nongenotoxic Mechanisms

Genotoxicity entails damage to DNA; this genetic lesion may cause a phenotypic change when one allele is altered. In the absence of efficient repair systems, a linear dose-response relationship without a threshold dose can be considered a characteristic of such a mechanism. This may account for the fact that genotoxic carcinogens are frequently active at low doses and are occasionally active after a single exposure. Such characteristics indicate a high degree of potential hazard upon human exposure.

Alternatively, the change in DNA may require alterations of multiple alleles or loci, in which case a multihit model best describes the mechanism and may imply a threshold dose. Also, even though a compound has the capacity to induce DNA damage, such a response may be produced only after levels of toxicity or cell damage are induced. Such an indirect mechanism may provide for a no-effect level. Thus, the risk assessment of genotoxic carcinogens should include very careful analysis of all of the factors that could give insight into the mechanisms operative in the animal model.

The concept of nongenotoxicity is operational, i.e., it describes the effects of the agent using current methodology. Concepts or terminology may need to be modified as new facts are revealed. Barrows and Shank (1981) proposed that some agents which appear nongenotoxic in genotoxicity tests may, in fact, induce genetic damage on administration to animals. They showed that toxic levels of hydrazine caused aberrant methylation of DNA to give O^6 and N^7 methylguanines, the methyl group having been derived from S-adenosyl methionine. This aberrant methylation apparently arises from chronic insult to the tissue and could underlie most of what appears to be nongenotoxic carcinogenicity. The extent of aberrant methylation involved in a carcinogenic response has not been determined, but if it is a mechanism of carcinogenesis, the terms "direct" and "indirect" genotoxicity may be more appropriate. Nevertheless, the overall concept would not be affected since aberrant methylation is apparently dependent on sustained chemical injury to the tissue. It has been speculated that a differential ability of C_3H and C57BL mice to synthesize methyltransferase in response to aberrant DNA methylation by intracellular methyl donors could be a mechanism explaining the differences between these mouse strains in incidences of spontaneous hepatocellular carcinoma (Lindamood et al., 1984).

Some nongenotoxic carcinogens, such as NTA, show an apparent threshold in the dose-response curve (Anderson et al., 1982). If the threshold is far beyond predicted human exposures, this may be a useful observation for risk assessment since a conventional toxicological safety factor may be applied in assessing a safe exposure level for man. The demonstration of such a threshold does not necessarily indicate that a carcinogen acts by a nongenotoxic mechanism. In the U.S. National Center for Toxicological Research's ED_{01} experiment (Society of Toxicology, 1981; Staffa and Mehlman, 1979) with the genotoxic carcinogen 2-AAF, the bladder tumors exhibited a no-observed effect level (NOEL) against a low background rate, while the liver tumors showed much less curvature in the dose-response relation (Hughes et al., 1983). Even with a study of this magnitude, however, a careful analysis of the liver tumor data has not completely ruled out the possibility of a threshold (Brown and Hoel, 1983).

Induced tumors which occur in the presence of an appreciable "spontaneous" background tumor incidence of the same cell type appear to yield linear dose-response curves. This is probably due to the fact that the carcinogen or promoter has only to accelerate the appearance of such tumors and not to affect the complex, multistage processes of complete carcinogenesis. Such an enhancement of tumor yield does not permit the genotoxic or nongenotoxic mode of action of the carcinogen to be directly assessed from the chronic animal bioassay. On the other hand, the induction of rare (infrequently occurring) tumors may indicate that the test chemical acts by a genotoxic mechanism (Clayson et al., 1983).

Chemical carcinogens exhibit a wide variety of biological effects (Section VII). Each of these effects should be considered in an effort to decide on the probable relevance of animal carcinogenicity to man and on the relative importance of the genotoxic and nongenotoxic elements of the mode of action. Decisions on possible human risk need to be made on a case-by-case basis. The criteria used must address the likelihood in man of all recognized biological effects demonstrated to be of probable importance in the induction of tumors. For example, present evidence suggests that diethylstilbestrol is a carcinogen in animals because of its estrogenic activity. Since it is estrogenic also in man, its lack of genotoxicity may be of little importance to human risk assessment. The estrogenic dose is then the important criterion since the effects are mediated through the hormonal action rather than through direct genotoxicity. NTA, on the other hand, requires massive doses administered to rats and mice in order to induce urinary tract tumors. This involves either disruption of ionic balances (Anderson *et al.*, 1982) or induction of physical trauma in the urinary tract epithelium. There are thresholds for these effects. Neither effect is conceivable at the level to which man is likely to be exposed.

It should, nevertheless, not be assumed *a priori* that because a carcinogen is nongenotoxic it is of lesser concern with respect to possible human health effects. Indeed, several of the major cancers may be attributable in large part to the effects of cancer-enhancing agents related to lifestyle factors (Doll and Peto, 1981; Gori, 1978; Weisburger and Williams, 1980). Risk assessment for nongenotoxic carcinogens is dependent on several discrete sequential decisions. First, the agent is demonstrated to be carcinogenic in animals. Second, the agent is shown to be lacking in genotoxic potential. Third, biological studies suggest a mechanism by which it is likely that the agent induces tumors. Fourth, it can be demonstrated that humans under predicted conditions of exposure are, or are not, likely to be affected in the same way as are experimental animals. The importance of the third and fourth considerations is illustrated by asbestos and TCDD, neither of which is genotoxic. Each may be involved in human exposure in quantities either sufficient to produce tumors (asbestos), or (taking into account high potency) likely to do so (TCDD). Thus the setting of realistic exposure limits for man is exceptionally difficult.

VII. Systematic Analysis of the Chemical and Biological Properties of Carcinogens

7.1. Introduction

Several authors (Grice, 1978; Health Council of the Netherlands, 1980; IRLG, 1979, 1980; Squire, 1981b; Stott *et al.*,, 1981; Weisburger and Williams, 1982, 1984; Williams, 1980a) have proposed multivariate schemes to assess the carcinogenic potential of chemicals in the evaluation of human health risks. The importance in making regulatory decisions of looking beyond tumor pathogenesis and considering the total weight of evidence on carcinogenicity has been stressed (Clayson *et al.*, 1983; Nutrition Foundation, 1983). The following section outlines several chemical and biological properties that should be considered in assessment of carcinogenic risk of chemicals to humans. None of these properties, taken individually, necessarily provide unequivocal evidence that a chemical is or is not a carcinogen. Rather, it is important to consider the cumulative weight of evidence for carcinogenicity derived from a judicious assessment of all of the properties of the substance.

7.2. Chemical

Chemical structure. Chemical structure may be of value in suggesting similarities to known carcinogens or in suggesting the likely way in which the agent will be metabolized (Asher and Zervos, 1977; Miller and Miller, 1976). In addition, the chemical structure can be analyzed for the presence of configurations known to give rise to electrophilic reactants. Such configurations would suggest potential genotoxicity. Chemical structure by itself, however, is an uncertain predictor of carcinogenic activity, since small changes in molecular structure within a class of carcinogens may greatly affect biological response. This is illustrated by carcinogen/noncarcinogen pairs such as benzo(a)pyrene and benzo(e)-pyrene or 3'-methyl-4-dimethylaminoazobenzene and 2-methyl-4-di-methylaminoazobenzene or 2,3,7,8-TCDD and 1,3,6,8-TCDD.

7.3. Biotransformation, Metabolism and Pharmacokinetics

Biotransformation. Most carcinogens undergo biotransformation leading to detoxification and, to a lesser degree, to metabolic activation (Miller and Miller, 1976; Weisburger and Williams, 1982). The ratio of activation to detoxification, that is, the proportion of the carcinogen that is converted to an effective form, varies widely. This variation occurs between species, with the stage of maturity of the test animals, with the dose of carcinogen, and with the presence of other chemicals such as enzyme-inducing agents.

Metabolism and pharmacokinetics. Information on metabolism and pharmacokinetics is needed for intra- and inter-species evaluation. Such information is useful in assessing the mechanism of action and the suitability of the test animal for extrapolation of the findings to humans. Metabolism data can explain qualitative and quantitative differences in potency. For example, nonlinear pharmacokinetics may indicate changes in the rates of biotransformation and disposition which may markedly alter the carcinogenic potency of a chemical (Gehring and Blau, 1977). The multiple genetic and environmental factors capable of affecting rates of carcinogen absorption, distribution, metabolism and excretion have been considered by Vesell (1980).

7.4. Biochemical Reactivity

Carcinogen interactions. Many carcinogens or their metabolites react with DNA to form covalent adducts. Benzo(a)pyrene metabolites form adducts with DNA bases (Grunberger and Weinstein, 1979; Jeffrey *et al.*, 1980), and activated aromatic amines attack the C-8 and N-2 positions of guanine (Beland *et al.*, 1983; Kreik and Westra, 1979). Alkylating agents can methylate or ethylate nitrogens or oxygens in DNA bases (Singer and Kroger, 1979). Aflatoxin epoxides attack the C-8 and N-2 positions of guanine (Lin *et al.*, 1977). Such adducts, or other forms of DNA damage, may lead to irreversible genetic change, i.e., genotoxicity (see Section III). Reactions with DNA may result in the induction of a tumorigenic phenotype either directly (through somatic mutation), or indirectly (by altering gene expression) (Radman *et al.*, 1977; Razin and Friedman, 1981). Carcinogenic metals not reacting directly with DNA have been shown to affect the fidelity of DNA synthesis *in vitro* (Loeb *et al.*, 1981). Other intracellular macromolecules may also be affected by the carcinogen or its active metabolites and this, too, may affect the carcinogenic process. The degree of adduct formation *in vivo* or *in vitro* may be useful in explaining potency differences (Booth *et al.*, 1981).

7.5. Host: Non-neoplastic Determinants

Relevant non-neoplastic functional effects in the host. This heading encompasses diverse effects such as: hormonal imbalance (IARC, 1974a), nutritional imbalance, stress, immune status changes (Baldwin, 1973; Kroes *et al.*, 1975; Prehn, 1973), or indirect effects resulting from physiologic changes (see Section 2.13). An example of the latter is achlorhydria, induced by H_2-receptor antagonist drugs. These drugs lead to bacterial overgrowth in the stomach and increased *in vivo* nitrosation of ingested chemicals (Hill, 1980).

Relevant non-neoplastic morphological effects. Data on these include qualitative and quantitative information on biochemical, pharmacological, physiological and morphological effects. An example of this is solid state carcinogenesis due to physical factors, such as the development of bladder stones with the subsequent development of bladder tumors. Other lesions relate to stress and include increases in the incidence of stress-associated gastric ulcers in rats, accelerated thymic atrophy, and altered severity of amyloidosis in mice. Such effects may give additional information regarding the pathogenesis of the neoplasia involved (Bischoff and Bryson, 1964; Brand, 1975; Casarett and Doull, 1975; Clarke, 1983; Clayson, 1975; Health Council of the Netherlands, 1980; Kroes, 1979; Schumann *et al.*, 1980; Stott *et al.*, 1981).

7.6. Host: Neoplastic Determinants

Species and strain specificity. Some carcinogens have marked species specificity. Bladder stones, for example, have the effect of readily inducing bladder tumors in mice but apparently lack this property in humans (Clayson, 1979). Other chemicals cause the induction of bladder stones in mice and rats but only induce bladder tumors in rats (Melnick *et al.*, 1984). Carcinogens which have been shown to be genotoxic generally produce tumors in a variety of species and strains. However, this is not necessarily always a satisfactory criterion for distinguishing between genotoxic and nongenotoxic. For example, estrogenic hormones and goitrogens affect many species and tissues through nongenotoxic mechanisms. Moreover, most carcinogens which are known to be active in man are also active in a variety of other species (IARC, 1980a). Exceptions to this rule are benzene and arsenic, neither of which has yet been shown to produce tumors in animals despite the epidemiologic evidence of their human carcinogenicity. Chemicals that are active only in a single species or strain are possibly epigenetic and have mechanisms of action which are not reproducible in other species; this is in contrast to the situation with genotoxic carcinogens (FSC, 1978; IARC, 1982; IRLG, 1979, 1980).

The variety of histogenetic sites at which tumors occur in the various species tested. Nongenotoxic carcinogens generally affect only a single tissue or a few tissues in a limited number of species whereas the occurrence of malignant tumors at a number of different sites in a number of species is characteristic of some genetically active carcinogens. 2-naphthylamine, for example, affects the urinary bladder in man, dog, rat, hamster and monkey. 2-AAF affects many tissues such as liver, breast, intestine, ear duct and bladder in rats, mice and other species. N-nitroso compounds similarly affect a wide range of tissues in many species, depending upon the size of the administered dose. Tetrachloroethylene is an example of a nongenotoxic carcinogen that induces only liver tumors in mice.

Histologic and biologic characteristics of tumors. Tumors exhibiting characteristics associated with malignant behavior generally provide more persuasive evidence for oncogenic potential (see Section II) than do benign tumors by themselves.

Latent period in relation to dose. Latent period may be determined by the time required for the clinical manifestation of the tumor, and may be more precisely determined by interim sacrifice procedures.

Carcinogens which have produced tumors in high yield after short exposure are usually of the genotoxic type (IARC, 1982, 1983). The relation which exists between dose and the time-to-appearance of tumors can be used, together with tumor incidence, as an indicator of carcinogenic potency (Clayson, 1983; IARC, 1982, 1983). Time-to-tumor appearance by itself, however, is not an adequate criterion for distinguishing the two classes of carcinogens.

Relationship to background tumor incidence. The induction of rare (infrequently observed) tumor types is often associated with genotoxic agents (IARC 1982, 1983). In contrast, a dose-related increase in incidence of tumor types that have a significant background incidence may indicate that the treatment substance is a carcinogen, or a carcinogenesis enhancer, or a promoter (Clayson, 1981). The induction of tumors against an appreciable background tumor incidence (the specific level needs to be defined) may indicate that a genotoxic or nongenotoxic carcinogen or a non-specific stimulation is involved. Such observations must be supported by additional data including genotoxicity tests before the test agent is classified. For example, it appears that in the ED_{01} experiment (Society of Toxicology, 1981; Staffa and Mehlman, 1979) 2-AAF stimulated the appearance of liver neoplasia and is genotoxic. Agents such as carbon tetrachloride appear to act *in vivo* through cytotoxicity and regeneration, and are nongenotoxic in tests for acute genotoxicity.

The promotion of certain tumors that have a high background incidence in animals is not necessarily relevant to human risk assessment, since such a high background does not occur in man. Consequently promotion or enhancement of such tumors in test animals would not be expected in humans.

Qualitative and quantitative aspects of dose-response relationships. Dose-response relationships are of importance since they may aid in defining the potency of a carcinogenic compound, and provide information both on the shape of the curve and the extent to which no-observed-effect levels can be described. Comparison of the observed dose-response relationships with pharmacokinetic, metabolic or non-neoplastic effects help to provide insight with respect to possible mechanisms of action. However, by itself, the nature of the dose-response curve cannot be used to separate genotoxic and nongenotoxic carcinogens since on occasion both may yield threshold-type curves.

7.7. Short-Term Tests

Short-term tests for genotoxicity. Short-term tests have important applications in the interpretation of a cancer bioassay. (See accompanying monograph on short-term tests.) Most short-term tests detect genotoxic effects (see Section III) and, therefore, provide information on the capacity of the chemical to interact with DNA. Thus, positive evidence of the production of genetic effects by a carcinogen would suggest that the underlying mechanism of the tumor induction may have involved somatic mutation or a similar event.

Since somatic mutation is a stochastic process which may occur at low levels of exposure, genetically-active carcinogens deserve a high degree of concern. Nonetheless, the correlation between genetic damage and carcinogenic potential is only operational and should be used as a working hypothesis (Miller *et al.*, 1978).

Tests for promotion. One of the mechanisms by which chemicals can result in an increase in tumors is through the process of promotion (see Section III).

Promotion results in the expression of the neoplastic phenotype in initiated cells and has been attributed to a number of different mechanisms. For carcinogens that do not cause genetic damage, particularly those with limited carcinogenic activity, promoting effects in appropriate initiation/promotion models may provide insight into the carcinogenic mechanism (Hecker *et al.*, 1982; Sivak, 1982; Slaga *et al.*, 1978). Some current hypotheses to explain promotion implicate cellular membranes as a critical target (Sivak, 1978; Sivak and Tu, 1980; Weinstein *et al.*, 1982). A consequence of membrane alteration by tumor promoters is the inhibition of intercellular communication (Trosko *et al.*, 1981). Therefore, activity in short-term tests for this effect (see Section 3.7) suggest a promoting action.

7.8. Human Studies

Epidemiology. In reviewing the IARC Monograph program, Tomatis *et al.* (1978) stressed the general scarcity of epidemiological studies, which are mainly confined to retrospective evidence. While some experimental variables can be controlled in animal bioassays, very few variables can be controlled in retrospective or prospective epidemiological studies, although statistical procedures are available which help to factor out these confounding effects. Epidemiological studies may only provide suggestive evidence for a link between a chemical or industrial process and carcinogenicity. This suggestive finding usually has to be supplemented with animal bioassays to identify the specific compound responsible for the observed carcinogenicity and its potency. Exceptions do exist, however.

Health surveillance for exposure to carcinogenic stimuli. Surveillance studies may include chromosomal studies, biochemical studies (e.g., blood sugar, clinical chemistry), and special studies (e.g., sperm counts, immunological techniques) to detect individual exposure to carcinogens (Montesano *et al.*, 1982). Tannenbaum and Skipper (1983) have reviewed possible approaches to quantifying total mutagenic exposure in a given individual. Measurement of protein adducts, DNA adducts and mutation may be employed to indicate the remote and recent history of an individual's exposure to genetically toxic substances. In this area, human studies provide the basis for establishing the relevance of animal models.

7.9. Overview

The elucidation of carcinogenic mechanisms is of major concern if sound regulation of chemicals found to be carcinogenic in animal studies is to be achieved. When an attempt is being made to define mechanisms, the distinction between genotoxic and nongenotoxic (or acutely genotoxic and chronically genotoxic) carcinogens contributes to the elucidation. However, the overall mechanistic classification depends on an in-depth consideration of the chemical/biological properties of the substances as has been outlined above. If realistic subclassification of carcinogens is to be achieved, it is vital that distinctions be made, the totality of effects of each individual chemical be considered, and that an attempt be made to assess the relevance of these effects to disease in the human population.

Initiation, which appears to be a genotoxic phenomenon, and promotion, which appears to be nongenotoxic, are two discrete phases of carcinogenesis that can be identified with reasonable confidence. Our efforts to identify agents as initiating or nongenotoxic (promoting) represents a classification of the two extremes of the overall effect of carcinogens. As it becomes more feasible to quantitate these aspects of carcinogenesis, it is highly probable that a range of carcinogens will be identified from those which are almost pure initiators to those which are almost pure promoters. Some chemicals would be found to have a combined function. Such information will enable regulators to predict much more accurately than is now possible the probable carcinogenic effect of such agents upon human exposure.

7.10. Examples

See The Appendix.

VIII. Establishing Human Exposure Guidelines

The ultimate objective of the preceding analyses is to encourage the judicious utilization of all pertinent data in defining mechanisms of toxicity. With respect to carcinogenicity, this involves looking beyond the increased incidence of tumors in animal studies to all the relevant chemical and biological properties of the test compound. This approach will provide for the establishment of sound guidelines for human exposure to chemicals.

In the past it has been assumed that if a chemical was shown to be carcinogenic in animals, this fact alone indicated it would be carcinogenic in man. This assumption is reflected in most current regulatory approaches whereby animal carcinogens are treated as if they would generally be at least of equal and perhaps of greater risk to man. However, it is now becoming widely recognized that not all chemical carcinogens act via a common mechanism of action and, thus, may not present the same risk to man. In light of the differences in the mode of action there exists a need to distinguish between different classes of carcinogens and to develop appropriate options for regulation (Clayson, 1983; Grice, 1978; Kroes, 1979; Nutrition Foundation, 1983; Squire, 1981; Weisburger and Williams, 1980).

As detailed in Section VII, animal carcinogens may be roughly classified in terms of their genotoxic potential. Genotoxic agents act by direct interaction with genetic material, leading to irreversible self-replicating lesions. Nongenotoxic agents may act by a variety of indirect mechanisms such as recurrent cytotoxicity, physical irritation, hormonal imbalances, alterations in immunological or nutritional status, enzyme modification, and increased stress. An important characteristic of genotoxic carcinogens is that, in theory, they have the potential to initiate DNA damage at any level of exposure. In practice, however, it is possible that there may be non-zero levels of exposure where the risk is infinitesimal due to dose kinetics and repair mechanisms. Equally important is the possibility of threshold effects for nongenotoxic agents which act through indirect mechanisms involving modifications of normal physiological functions.

This distinction is of fundamental importance in terms of its implications for human risk assessment. Future policies on carcinogen regulation thus need to reflect the fact that chemicals of low carcinogenic potency which appear to induce tumors by virtue of their ability to cause physiological, toxicological or biochemical perturbations at high doses should possibly not be considered as hazardous as those clear-cut genotoxic agents that produce an abundance of tumors at low doses (Williams and Weisburger, 1981). At present, however, genotoxicity testing cannot be regarded as a foolproof way to distinguish between high and low risk animal carcinogens (Marshall, 1982). This is due to difficulties in unequivocally establishing whether or not a chemical is genotoxic (ICPEMC, 1983), and the fact that other related mechanisms of initiation need to be considered (Barrows and Shank, 1981). It also should be noted that promoting agents, devoid of detectable genotoxic action, may vary tremendously in potency, ranging from 2,3,7,8-TCDD on one end of the spectrum (Kociba et al., 1978) to saccharin at the other.

Traditionally, acceptable levels of exposure to compounds which induce toxic effects other than cancer have been established by the application of a suitable safety factor to the NOEL in animal studies. This approach is based on the fact that effects will be induced only when the level of exposure exceeds a certain critical level. The prediction of the critical level for man is the difficult problem. Considerations of sample size notwithstanding, the safety factor should take into account both intra- and inter-species differences in susceptibility in order to protect all segments of the population. The actual magnitude of the safety factor may also be influenced by the quality and scope of the available toxicological data.

To the extent possible, carcinogens have in the past been regulated in accordance with a zero-risk or zero-exposure principle which is consistent with a presumed absence of threshold effects for such compounds. A more recent approach to carcinogen regulation, which allows for options other than that dictated by the zero-risk principle, is the establishment of exposure guidelines which ensure that a minimal-risk level will not be exceeded. Although absolute safety cannot be demonstrated or assured in this case, a virtually safe dose corresponding to some suitably low level of risk may still be determined. This may be done via extrapolation of experimental data downwards to the low dose region of interest (Brown and Koziol, 1983).

In view of these different possible strategies for regulating different types of carcinogenic agents, it is important to establish criteria which may be used to evaluate genotoxic potential. The chemical properties of the test compound such as similarity to known carcinogens, electrophilic characteristics, or ability to interact with DNA may assist in defining the type of carcinogen involved and its mechanism of action. In general, the carcinogenicity bioassay in small rodents provides information as to the carcinogenic potential of the test agent but not on its mechanism of action. A properly conducted bioassay will, however, provide much information on the dose-response characteristics of the chemical and its corresponding potency in the animal species used. The spectrum of neoplasia in the various tissues and organs as well as the number of species and strains affected also gives valuable information as to the level of concern. Non-neoplastic responses in the host can provide useful information in helping to define mechanisms.

A major piece of evidence as to the mechanism of action is provided by the short-term tests discussed in Section III. Most of these tests are designed to detect specific effects on genetic material such as somatic mutation, unscheduled DNA synthesis, chromosomal aberrations or SCE, and are, therefore, of great value in the identification of genotoxic agents. More recently, other short-term tests which focus on promotional effects have been proposed (Sivak, 1982). In addition to *in vitro* systems such as metabolic cooperation and possibly cell transformation assays, *in vivo* systems such as the altered development of lung adenomas and mammary tumors in certain rodent strains have been proposed. Although these systems require further validation, they offer considerable promise for the establishment of promotional effects and no-effect levels.

A careful assessment of both the long-term bioassay and short-term test data may provide a means of distinguishing between compounds with genotoxic properties and those which act by other means. A systematic analysis of other chemical and biological characteristics of the compound may provide additional information as to the likelihood of threshold effects and possible mechanisms. Exposure guidelines for the compounds for which the threshold hypothesis appears plausible may then be determined through the application of a suitable safety factor. This should take into account all of the available data as well as an accounting of the population at risk. For compounds considered to present some small elevation in risk even at very low levels of exposure, the notion of absolute safety may be replaced by that of virtual safety. Because of the uncertainties as to the shape of experimental dose-response curves in the low dose region, some forms of linear extrapolation may be employed in an attempt to obtain an upper limit in the low dose risk.

IX. Appendix: Profiles of Selected Compounds

This appendix consists of a summary of the chemical and biological properties of selected compounds which exhibit some degree of carcinogenic activity in test animals. The purpose of this compendium is to illustrate how the available chemical and biological data on a variety of compounds may be presented in summary form. The summaries are useful for a quick review of pertinent data and for identification of missing data.

2-AMINOFLUORENE (2AF)

I. CHEMICAL

1. Chemical Structure

> *Similarity to known carcinogens.* One of many polycyclic aromatic amine carcinogens (Clayson and Garner, 1976). 2AF and some of its metabolites induce tumors.

> *Reactivity.* Not reactive unless activated (Clayson and Garner, 1976; Weisburger and Williams, 1982).

2. Biotransformation and Pharmacokinetics

> Acetylation and N-hydroxylation followed by further transformation to reactive derivatives (Clayson and Garner, 1976; Miller, 1978; Weisburger and Williams, 1982).

> Most metabolism performed by cytoplasmic enzymes, but nuclear enzymes also involved (Kawarjiri *et al.*, 1979).

3. Biochemical Reactivity

Following metabolism undergoes covalent interaction with proteins and nucleic acids. The covalent adducts in DNA occur on guanine (Kriek and Wetra, 1979; Sake *et al.*, 1978; Stout *et al.*, 1980; Takeishi *et al.*, 1979).

II. HOST NON-NEOPLASTIC EFFECTS

1. Relevant Functional Effects in the Host

Increase in P-448, smooth and rough endoplasmic reticulum (Okita, 1976; Pooke and Parke, 1978).

2. Relevant Non-neoplastic Morphologic Effects

Acetylated derivative produces pre-neoplastic altered foci in rat liver within 3 weeks (Williams and Watanabe, 1978). Hyperplasia of bladder transitional epithelium develops as early as one week (Frith and Jaques, 1974).

III. HOST NEOPLASTIC DETERMINANTS

1. Species and Strains Tested

Mouse, rat (Clayson and Garner, 1976).

2. Variety of Histogenetic Tumor Sites in Species Tested

Mouse: liver, possibly bladder;
Rat: liver, mammary gland, intestine, ear duct (Miller *et al.*, 1964; Weisburger and Weisburger, 1958; Weisburger, 1964).

3. Histologic and Biologic Characteristics of Tumors

High proportion of malignant tumors in all affected tissues (Miller *et al.*, 1964; Weisburger and Weisburger, 1958).

4. Latent Period in Relation to Dose

Less than one year for liver tumors in rats.

5. Relationship to Background Tumor Incidence

Increased liver and mammary gland background incidence in rats, but also produces tumors with low spontaneous occurrence.

6. Qualitative and Quantitative Aspects of Dose-response Relationships

No information available.

IV. SHORT-TERM TESTS

1. Short-Term Tests for Genotoxicity

Mutagenicity

Bacteria	pos.	(McCann *et al.*, 1975)
Mammalian cells	pos.	(Clive *et al.*, 1979)
Drosophila	pos.	(Vogel *et al.*, 1980)

Chromosomal aberrations

Human lymphocytes	pos.	(Williams, 1981a)
DNA repair synthesis	pos.	(Williams, 1981b)
Sister chromatid exchange	pos.	(Schreck, 1979)
Cell transformation	pos.	(Pienta, 1980)

2. Tests for Promotion

No information available.

V. HUMAN STUDIES

1. Epidemiology

No information available.

2. Health Surveillance

No information available.

VI. SUMMARY

2AF induces a variety of tumors in both mice and rats. It undergoes metabolic activation to an electrophilic species which binds to DNA and is active in a variety of short-term tests for genotoxicity. 2AF is thus a clear genotoxic carcinogen.

BENZENE

I. CHEMICAL

1. Chemical Structure

Similarity to known carcinogens. 1,2 benzenedicarbonitril.

IX. Appendix: Profiles of Selected Compounds

Reactivity. No information available.

2. Biotransformation and Pharmacokinetics

Excretion. Benzene is exhaled unchanged in expired air (dog, rat, mouse, rabbit, man) (Andrews *et al.*, 1977; Parke and Williams, 1953; Rickert *et al.*, 1979; Schreck *et al.*, 1941).

Metabolism. Benzene → benzeneoxide → phenol → 1,2,3, and 4:
  1. → (glutathione) → premercapturic acid
  2. → (epoxide hydratase) → 1,2-benzenediol → catechol
  3. → (?) → hydroquinone
  4. other, among others trihydroxylated benzene, muconic acid
   (Snyder *et al.*, 1981)

Metabolites excreted mainly as sulfates or glucuronides. Metabolism in liver stimulated by enzyme inducing agents. Benzene is a myelotoxic compound (Longacre *et al.*, 1980, 1981a, 1981b).

3. Biochemical Reactivity

C^{14} labelled benzene shows covalent binding with proteins from liver, bone marrow, kidney, lung, spleen, blood and muscle *in vitro* and also binds to the nuclear fraction of bone marrow cells (Irons *et al.*, 1980; Longacre *et al.*, 1980, 1981a, 1981b; Snyder *et al.*, 1978a).

II. HOST NON-NEOPLASTIC EFFECTS

1. Relevant Functional Effects in the Host

Myelotoxic, effect on reproduction, teratogenic (IARC, 1982).

2. Relevant Non-neoplastic Morphologic Effects

Leukopenia, anemia, thrombocytopenia, aplastic anemia, immunosuppressive in CFU-formation in bone marrow and spleen (IARC, 1982).

III. HOST NEOPLASTIC DETERMINANTS

1. Species and Strains Tested

Rat (Sprague-Dawley)
Mice (57BL/6) (Charles River CD1)

2. Variety of Histogenetic Tumor Sites in Species Tested

Tumors	Dose per mg/kg bw		
	0	50(x)	250(x)
Female: Zymbal's gland	0/30	2/30	8/32
Female: mammary carcinomas	3/30	4/30	7/32
Female: leukemia	1/30	2/30	1/21
Male: leukemia	0/30	0/30	4/33

(x) by stomach tube 4–5 days weekly, 52 weeks

Skin. Negative results: no tumors (Burdette and Strong, 1941; Coombs and Croft, 1966; Fukuda *et al*., 1981; Kirschbaum and Strong, 1942; Laerum, 1973; Neukomm, 1962).

Inhalation. No dose-response in mice studies. Lympho- and/or hematopoietic system at levels of 300 ppm (900 mg/m^3: 8/40 mice versus 2/40 controls (Snyder *et al*., 1980), 2/40 mice (Snyder *et al*., 1978a). No tumors in rats (300 ppm) (Snyder *et al*., 1978b).

Subcutaneous. In various studies in mice, in which only one dose was tested, an increase (not significant) in hematopoietic or lympho-poietic tumors was noticed (Amiel, 1960; Ward *et al*., 1975).

3. Histologic and Biologic Characteristics of Tumors

Not studied.

4. Latent Period in Relation to Dose

No information available.

5. Relationship to Background Tumor Incidence

In the carcinogenicity studies tumors of the lympho- and/or hematopoietic system occurred in the controls in low incidences. (see 2)

6. Qualitative and Quantitative Aspects of Dose-response Relationships

Some indication of dose-response in one study in rats (Maltoni and Scarnato, 1979), but essentially data are insufficient.

IV. SHORT-TERM TESTS

1. Short-Term Tests for Genotoxicity

Mutagenicity

Prokaryotic systems:

Bacteria	Neg.	(Cotruvo *et al.*, 1977; Dean, 1978; IARC, 1976a; Lebowitz *et al.*, 1978; Tanooka, 1977)
Yeast	Neg.	(Rosenkranz and Leifer, 1980; Shahin and Fournier, 1978)
Mammalian cells	Neg.	(Lebowitz *et al.*, 1978)
Drosophila	Neg.	(Nylander *et al.*, 1978)

Chromosomal aberrations	Pos.	(possibly due to biologically active metabolites rather than benzene itself), (Gerner-Smidt and
	Neg.	Friedrich, 1978; Koizumi *et al.*, 1974; Morimoto, 1976)
Micronucleus	Pos.	(Diaz *et al.*, 1980; Hite *et al.*, 1980; IARC, 1976a)

Sister chromatid exchange	Neg.	(Diaz *et al.*, 1979; Morimoto and Wolff, 1980)

Germ cell effects

Dominant lethal	Neg.	(IARC, 1976a)

2. Tests for Promotion

No information available.

V. HUMAN STUDIES

1. Epidemiology

Chronic human exposure to benzene results in leukopenia, anemia, thrombocytopenia or combinations of these. A clear correlation between benzene exposure and chromosomal aberration in bone marrow and peripheral lymphocytes has been found in individuals exposed to high levels of benzene (> 100 ppm). Several case-control studies as well as cohort studies showed significant association between leukemia (predominantly myelogenous) and occupational exposure to various solvents including benzene. Two follow-up studies showed high incidences of leukemia ascertained as cases of benzene hemopathy (IARC, 1982).

2. Health Surveillance

(See 1)

VI. SUMMARY

In humans a significant association has been found between exposure to benzene and leukemia. Benzene caused tumors in rats after oral administration and in mice after subcutaneous administration but not necessarily of the hematopoietic system. In short-term genotoxicity tests benzene was negative whereas *in vivo* positive results were obtained in the micronucleus test. It shows covalent binding with protein, is an immunosuppressant, and is myelotoxic. Although benzene is strongly suspected as a human carcinogen at relatively high exposure levels, the experimental evidence in rodents is not conclusive. Benzene is not genotoxic; an indirect carcinogenic action involving myelotoxic action is likely but should be further elucidated.

CHLOROFORM

I. CHEMICAL

1. Chemical Structure

Similarity to known carcinogens. Chloroform is a small halogenated hydrocarbon. Many halogenated hydrocarbons have been found to induce liver tumors in mice when tested in the National Cancer Institute bioassays.

Reactivity. Oxidized by strong oxidizing agents such as chromic acid, with formation of phosgene and chlorine gas; reacts with halogens or halogenating agents; reacts with primary amines to form isonitriles; reacts with phenols in alkaline solution to form hydroxy-substituted aromatic aldehydes; relatively unreactive in aqueous media at physiological pH and room temperature (IARC, 1979a).

2. Biotransformation and Pharmacokinetics

Pohl (1979) reviewed the biochemical toxicology of chloroform and concluded that its toxicity was related to its metabolic transformation to reactive intermediates. This is consistent with the increased toxicity of chloroform in animals previously treated with inducers of mixed function oxidases and the decreased toxicity of chloroform in animals treated with inhibitors of mixed function oxidases. Pohl *et al.* (1977) concluded that the toxicity of chloroform was related to the production of phosgene intermediates rather than the production of free radicals such as seem to occur for carbon tetrachloride.

Chloroform appears to be rapidly eliminated from the body of exposed animals. Primary routes are exhalation and metabolism to materials excreted in the urine (Pohl, 1979). There appears to be little potential for bioaccumulation of chloroform, and metabolism appears to be most extensive in the smaller animal species, making them more susceptible to the toxicity of chloroform (Reitz *et al.*, 1978).

3. Biochemical Reactivity

Covalent binding of chloroform to tissue macromolecules (primarily protein) has been demonstrated *in vivo* and *in vitro* (Illett *et al.*, 1973). *In vivo* binding of chloroform to DNA, however, is very low (Reitz *et al.*, 1980a).

Free radical formation has not been demonstrated for chloroform *in vivo*. Instead the primary pathways for metabolism appear to involve phosgene (Pohl *et al.*, 1977).

II. HOST NON-NEOPLASTIC EFFECTS

1. Relevant Functional Effects in the Host

Physiological: Renal function impaired in male mice.
Pharmacological: Narcotizing at higher doses (Pohl, 1979).
Biochemical: Depletes liver glutathione (Pohl, 1979).

2. Relevant Non-neoplastic Morphologic Effects

Fatty degeneration of liver in rats; frank necrosis in liver of rats; severe kidney damage in male mice; liver damage in humans following very high doses (Pohl, 1979).

III. HOST NEOPLASTIC DETERMINANTS

1. Species and Strains Tested

Positive in rats and mice, with mice much more sensitive than rats (NCI, 1976); positive in one strain of mouse (four tested) and negative in rats and dogs (Heywood *et al.*, 1979; Palmer *et al.*, 1979; Roe *et al.*, 1979).

2. Variety of Histogenetic Tumor Sites in Species Tested

Liver and kidney in male mice; liver in female mice; kidney in male rats.

3. Histologic and Biologic Characteristics of Tumors

Mixture of benign and malignant tumors.

4. Latent Period in Relation to Dose

No information available.

5. Relationship to Background Tumor Incidence

Increases a relatively high rate of spontaneous liver tumors in mice. Increases the rate of kidney tumors in rats and one strain of mouse (four tested). Kidney tumors do occur spontaneously in rats and mice, but much less frequently than liver tumors.

6. Qualitative and Quantitative Aspects of Dose-response Relationships

Appears to be a no-effect level for tumorigenicity of chloroform.

IV. SHORT-TERM TESTS

1. Short-Term Tests for Genotoxicity

Mutagenicity

Bacteria	neg.	(de Serres and Ashby, 1981b; Van Abbé *et al.*, 1982)
Yeast	neg.	(Bridges *et al.*, 1981; Uehleke *et al.*, 1977)
DNA repair synthesis	neg.	(Brookes and Preston, 1981)
Sister chromatic exchange	neg.	(Brookes and Preston, 1981)
Cell transformation	neg.	(Brookes and Preston, 1981)

2. Tests for Promotion

No information available.

V. HUMAN STUDIES

1. Epidemiology

No history of increased tumor incidence in chronically exposed (up to 10 years) confectionery workers.

2. Health Surveillance

No information available.

VI. SUMMARY

Chloroform causes a mixture of benign and malignant liver and kidney tumors in some strains of mice and rats and is negative in others. It is negative in a wide variety of short-term tests for genotoxicity. Although chloroform binds with macromolecules to some degree, no evidence of adduct formation is available. While it causes severe tissue damage in both liver and kidney and appears to be nongenotoxic, the precise mechanism of action is unclear.

CHLORDANE

I. CHEMICAL

1. Chemical Structure

Similarity to known carcinogens. One of several carcinogenic halogenated polycyclic aromatic hydrocarbons (Williams, 1981a).

Reactivity. Highly lipophilic.

2. Biotransformation and Pharmacokinetics

3. Biochemical Reactivity

Carcinogen interaction.

II. HOST NON-NEOPLASTIC EFFECTS

1. Relevant Functional Effects in the Host

Induces cytochrome P-450 and drug metabolizing enzymes (Madhukar and Matsumura, 1979; Stenger *et al.*, 1975).

2. Relevant Non-neoplastic Morphologic Effects

Increase smooth endoplasmic reticulum (Stenger *et al.*, 1975).

III. HOST NEOPLASTIC DETERMINANTS

1. Species and Strains Tested

Rats: Osborne Mendel (NCI, 1977a).
Mice: $B6C3F_1$

2. Variety of Histogenetic Tumor Sites in Species Tested

Only liver tumors, only in mice (NCI, 1977a).

3. Histologic and Biologic Characteristics of Tumors

Mouse liver tumors: ratio of benign to malignant is 1:10 (NCI, 1977a).

4. Latent Period in Relation to Dose

Liver tumors in mice about 60 weeks (NCI, 1977a).

5. Relationship to Background Tumor Incidence

Spontaneous liver tumors in B6C3F$_1$ mice used for bioassay.

6. Qualitative and Quantitative Aspects of Dose-response Relationships

In mice, 30 and 60 ppm both produce liver tumors (NCI, 1977a). In male and female Osborne Mendel rats, 400 and 250 ppm negative (NCI, 1977a).

IV. SHORT-TERM TESTS

1. Short-Term Tests for Genotoxicity

Mutagenicity

Bacteria	neg.	(Ashwood-Smith *et al.*, 1972)
Mammalian cells		
V79	pos.	(Ahmed *et al.*, 1977a)
Liver epithelial	neg.	(Telang *et al.*, 1982; Williams, 1980b)
HeLa cells	neg.	(Brandt *et al.*, 1972)
DNA repair synthesis	neg.	(Griffin and Hill, 1978)

Germ cell effects

Dominant lethal mouse	neg.	(Arnold *et al.*, 1977)
Chromosomal aberrations	pos.	(Ahmed *et al.*, 1977b)

2. Tests for Promotion

Inhibits intracellular communication between cultured liver cells (Telang *et al.*, 1982).

V. HUMAN STUDIES

1. Epidemiology

No information available.

2. Health Surveillance

No information available.

VI. SUMMARY

Chlordane induces malignant liver tumors in male and female mice, but is noncarcinogenic in rats. This compound is inactive in a number of different short-term tests for genotoxicity. There are two unconfirmed positive results from one laboratory, and one positive result in an *in vitro* test for promotion. Chlordane belongs to the class of halogenated polycyclic aromatic hydrocarbons which are principally hepatocarcinogenic in mice. It is thus considered to be a nongenotoxic agent, probably operating as a promoter.

CLOFIBRATE

I. CHEMICAL

1. Chemical Structure

Similarity to known carcinogens. Some other hypolipidemic agents (Reddy *et al.*, 1980).

Reactivity. No information available.

2. Biotransformation and Pharmacokinetics

Effects are on triglyceride levels, lipid and cholesterol synthesis.

3. Biochemical Reactivity

Does not interact with or cause damage to DNA (Warren *et al.*, 1980).

II. HOST NON-NEOPLASTIC EFFECTS

1. Relevant Functional Effects in the Host

Rats. Initial response liver enlargement proliferation of smooth endoplasmic reticulum, increase in peroxisomes alterations in peroxisome structure and peroxisome enzyme activity.
Hamsters, dogs, mice. Increase in peroxisomes (Barnard *et al.*, 1979; Elek and Jambor, 1978; Hess *et al.*, 1965; Schwandt *et al.*, 1978).
Monkeys. No increase in peroxisomes (IARC, 1980a; Svoboda and Azarnoff, 1979).

Man. No evidence of peroxisome proliferation. Increase in smooth endoplasmic reticulum and mitochondria, no cellular damage (de la Iglesia and Farber, 1983; Hanefeld *et al.*, 1977, 1980; Reddy and Rao, 1977).

Cohen and Grasso (1981) suggested that the bioavailability of catalase in the liver peroxisomes of rodents treated with clofibrate is insufficient to cope with the detoxification of injurious H_2O_2 concentrations resulting from the considerably enhanced activity of H_2O_2-generating enzymes. Liver cells may thus be exposed to the cytotoxic or DNA-damaging potential as a result of the breakdown in homeostasis and such exposure could lead to the subsequent development of neoplasia in the rodent liver. It has also been postulated that liver carcinogenesis is linked to the endogenous metabolic disturbance(s) emanating from sustained increase in hepatic peroxisome population (Reddy *et al.*, 1980, 1982b; Warren *et al.*, 1980). On this premise it was suggested that there was an excess of endogenous H_2O_2 production in the liver of rats fed peroxisome proliferators thereby initiating carcinogenesis (Lalwani *et al.*, 1983).

2. Relevant Non-neoplastic Morphologic Effects

No frank histologic evidence of damage. Early subcellular liver change, i.e., smooth endoplasmic reticulum proliferation, peroxisome increase (Barnard *et al.*, 1980; Hanefeld *et al.*, 1977, 1980).

III. HOST NEOPLASTIC DETERMINANTS

1. Species and Strains Tested

Mice (Anon., 1981).
Rats: F344 (Reddy and Qureshi, 1979; Reddy and Rao, 1977; Svoboda and Azarnoff, 1979).

2. Variety of Histogenetic Tumor Sites in Species Tested

Liver (Reddy and Qureshi, 1979; Reddy and Rao, 1977; Svoboda and Azarnoff, 1979).

3. Histologic and Biologic Characteristics of Tumors

In rats mainly malignant; hepatocellular carcinomas only (Reddy and Qureshi, 1979; Reddy and Rao, 1977; Svoboda and Azarnoff, 1979).

4. Latent Period in Relation to Dose

Over six months (Reddy and Qureshi, 1979; Reddy and Rao, 1977; Svoboda and Azarnoff, 1979).

5. Relationship to Background Tumor Incidence

No increase over controls in C57BL/10J mice dosed up to 350 mg/ kg for 18 months (Anon., 1981).

6. Qualitative and Quantitative Aspects of Dose-response Relationships

Sharp increases over a narrow dose range. 350 mg/kg in rats. Not seen in two mouse studies at doses up to 350 mg/kg/day (Reddy and Qureshi, 1979; Reddy and Rao, 1977; Svoboda and Azarnoff, 1979).

IV. SHORT-TERM TESTS

1. Short-Term Tests for Genotoxicity

Mutagenicity

Bacteria	neg.	(Warren *et al.*, 1980)
DNA repair synthesis	neg.	(Warren *et al.*, 1980)

2. Tests for Promotion

Farber-Solt GGT assay under various regimens was negative (de la Iglesia and Farber, 1981).

V. HUMAN STUDIES

1. Epidemiology

Epidemiology studies have failed to reveal any excess liver cancer risk in clofibrate-treated patients (IARC, 1980a).

2. Health Surveillance

No information available.

VI. SUMMARY

Clofibrate induces hepatocellular carcinomas in rats, but is negative in mice. It does not cause damage to DNA and is negative in bacterial short-term tests for genotoxicity or initiation/promotion. At present, it is believed that the increase in peroxisomes contributes to hepatocarcinogenesis, possibly via nongenotoxic mechanisms of action. Evidence is accumulating that hypolipidemic drugs do not elicit peroxisome proliferative response in humans.

DICHLORODIPHENYLTRICHLOROETHANE (DDT)

I. CHEMICAL

1. Chemical Structure

Similarity to known carcinogens. One of a number of aromatic organochlorine compounds that produce rodent liver tumors (Williams, 1981a).

Reactivity. No information available.

2. Biotransformation and Pharmacokinetics

Dechlorinated to two principal metabolites, DDD and DDE, and through a series of intermediates to DDA (Peterson and Robinson, 1964). One of the metabolites, a chloro-olefin DDMU, has been postulated to be metabolized to a reactive epoxide (Gold *et al.*, 1981; Planche *et al.*, 1979).

3. Biochemical Reactivity

None

II. HOST NON-NEOPLASTIC EFFECTS

1. Relevant Functional Effects in Host

Pharmacological. Neurotoxic.

Biochemical. DDT is a non-competitive inhibitor of membrand (Na^+ K^+ and Ca^{2+} Mg^{2+}) ATPase (Price, 1975; Schneider, 1975).

Induces proliferation of smooth endoplasmic reticulum and increased activity of mixed function oxidases (Durham *et al.*, 1963; Hart and Fauts, 1963; Madhukar and Matsumura, 1979).

2. Relevant Non-neoplastic Morphologic Effects

No information available.

III. HOST NEOPLASTIC DETERMINANTS

1. Species and Strains Tested

   Produces liver tumors in mice (Kashyap *et al.*, 1977; Terracini *et al.*, 1973; Tomatis *et al.*, 1972; Turusov *et al.*, 1973) and rats (Rossi *et al.*, 1977) but not hamsters (Agthe *et al.*, 1970; Cabral *et al.*, 1980).

2. Variety of Histogenetic Tumor Sites in Species Tested

   Almost exclusively liver (IARC, 1979a; Williams, 1981d).

3. Histologic and Biologic Characteristics of Tumors

   Predominantly benign (IARC, 1979a).

4. Latent Period in Relation to Dose

   Mice. At dose of 100 ppm, tumors seen at 16 months (Walker *et al.*, 1973).

5. Relationship to Background Tumor Incidence

   Increased background incidence of liver tumors.

6. Qualitative and Quantitative Aspects of Dose-response Relationships

   Demonstrated to be a liver tumor promoter (Nishizumi, 1979; Peraino *et al.*, 1975, 1980).

IV. SHORT-TERM TESTS

1. Short-Term Tests for Genotoxicity

   Mutagenicity

Bacteria	neg.	(Marshall *et al.*, 1976; Planche *et al.*, 1979; Van Dijck and Van de Voorde, 1976)
Yeast	neg.	(Fahring, 1974)
Insect	neg.	(Grosch and Valcovic, 1967)
Rat liver epithelial cells	neg.	(Williams, 1979b)
Human fibroblasts	neg.	(Tong *et al.*, 1981)
Mice	neg.	(Epstein and Shafer, 1968; Wallace, 1976)

DNA damage

DNA-protein linking	pos.	(Kubinski *et al.*, 1981)
DNA binding	neg.	(Griffin and Hill, 1978)
Hepatocyte DNA repair	neg.	(Maslansky and Williams, 1981; Probst *et al.*, 1981)
Fibroblast DNA repair	neg.	(Ahmed *et al.*, 1977b)

Chromosome effects

Human lymphocytes	neg.	(Lessa *et al.*, 1976)

2. Tests for Promotion

Demonstrated to be a liver tumor promoter (Nishizumi, 1979; Peraino *et al.*, 1975, 1980). A positive inhibitor of intercellular communication (Williams *et al.*, 1981).

V. HUMAN STUDIES

1. Epidemiology

No evidence of human carcinogenicity (Deichmann and Mac-Donald, 1977; IARC, 1979a).

2. Health Surveillance

Biomedical monitoring. DDT is accumulated in several tissues including liver and adipose tissue (Egan *et al.*, 1965; Hattula *et al.*, 1976; Morgan and Roan, 1971).

VI. SUMMARY

DDT produces predominantly benign liver tumors in some species of mice but not in others. It causes similar lesions in rats but not in hamsters. It is negative in many short-term tests for genotoxicity, does not bind to DNA, but inhibits intercellular communication among liver cells. Tumor-promoting activity has also been demonstrated in liver. It is a member of the class of halogenated polycyclic aromatic hydrocarbons and appears to be a nongenotoxic liver tumor promoter.

ETHYLENE THIOUREA (ETU)

I. CHEMICAL

1. Chemical Structure

   Similarity to known carcinogens. Some other anti-thyroid agents, e.g., carbamyl, thiocarbamyl, thiourea and thioacetamide (IARC, 1976b).

   Reactivity. No information available.

2. Biotransformation and Pharmacokinetics

   Rats. Single dose 4 mg/kg of ^{14}C ETU is eliminated within 24 hours; 1/2t 5-6 hours-62.6% unchanged. Imidazolone, imidazoline and ethylene urea are metabolites (Iverson *et al.*, 1980).

3. Biochemical Reactivity

   High doses of ETU administered by i.p. injection, nasogastric intubation or in food failed to inhibit the synthesis of nuclear or cytoplasmic RNA (Austin and Moyer, 1979).

II. HOST NON-NEOPLASTIC EFFECTS

1. Relevant Functional Effects in the Host

   125 ppm caused decreases in serum triiodothyronine and thyroxine and marked increases in thyroid stimulating hormone (TSH) levels (Blackwell-Smith *et al.*, 1953). ^{131}I was significantly decreased in male rats fed ETU in the diet for 12, 18 or 24 months (Graham *et al.*, 1975).

2. Relevant Non-neoplastic Morphologic Effects

   90 days, 125 ppm, thyroid. Marked hyperplasia of lining cells with microfollicular follicles and absence of colloid. Increased thyroid weight. Liver–central zone–increased cytoplasm fewer nuclei– less orderly hepatic cords (Blackwell-Smith *et al.*, 1953; Graham *et al.*, 1973, 1975; Ulland *et al.*, 1972).

III. HOST NEOPLASTIC DETERMINANTS

1. Species and Strains Tested

   Mice: (1) C57BL/6xC3H/Anf F$_1$
          (2) C57BL/6xAKR F$_1$ (IARC, 1974b)
   Rats: Charles River CD (Graham *et al.*, 1973, 1975)

2. Variety of Histogenetic Tumor Sites in Species Tested

			ETU	Control
Mice Hepatoma	(1)	male	14/16	8/79
		female	18/18	0/87
				(IARC, 1974b)
Rats Charles River CD				
Thyroid	(2)	male	18/18	5/90
		female	9/16	1/82
				(Graham et al.,
				1973, 1975)

Severity and extent of reversibility of the histopathological lesions were found to be a function of the duration of exposure to ETU (Arnold et al., 1982).

3. Histologic and Biologic Characteristics of Tumors

Benign and malignant thyroid tumors.

4. Latent Period in Relation to Dose

Thyroid carcinoma in female rats at 68 weeks.

5. Relationship to Background Tumor Incidence

Hepatoma in mice. Increased incidence over controls (IARC, 1974b).
Thyroid follicular cell tumors in rats. Increased incidence of adenoma and carcinoma over control (Graham et al., 1975).

6. Qualitative and Quantitative Aspects of Dose-response Relationships

Rats fed dietary levels of 125 ppm for 12 months had thyroid hyperplasia. Some carcinoma in rats fed 250 ppm. Rats were fed 175 or 350 ppm in diet for 18 months followed by administration of control diet for 6 months. Mice 215 mg/kg bw daily in gelatin by stomach tube (Graham et al., 1973, 1975).

Level of ETU in diet (ppm) (Graham et al., 1975)

Thyroid histopathology	0	5	25	125	250	500
Thyroid follicular cell carcinoma/adenocarcinoma	2	2	1	2	16	62

Thyroid histopathology	0	5	25	125	250	500
Thyroid follicular cell adenoma(s)	2	—	5	1	21	3
Thyroid follicular cell hyperplasia	4	20	41	44	27	3

IV. SHORT-TERM TESTS

1. Short-Term Tests for Genotoxicity

Mutagenicity

Bacteria	neg.	(Saffiotti *et al.*, 1979)
	weak pos.	(Schupbach and Hummler, 1977; Teramoto *et al.*, 1977)
Drosophila	neg.	(Mollet, 1975; Valencia and Houtchens, 1981)

Mammalian cells

In vitro Chinese hamster	neg.	(Teramoto *et al.*, 1977)
Human cell cultures	neg.	(Diala *et al.*, 1980)

Chromosomal aberrations

In vivo rat bone marrow	neg.	(Teramoto *et al.*, 1977)
Chinese hamster bone marrow	pos.	(Sram and Benes, 1974)
Micronucleus	neg.	(Schupbach and Hummler, 1977)

Germ cell effects

Dominant lethal	neg.	(Schupbach and Hummler, 1977; Sram and Benes, 1974; Teramoto *et al.*, 1977)
Mouse sperm abnormality	neg.	(Wyrobek *et al.*, 1981)

Sister chromatid exchange	neg.	(Paika *et al.*, 1981)
DNA repair synthesis	neg.	(Seiler, 1977)

2. Tests for Promotion

No information available.

V. HUMAN STUDIES

1. Epidemiology

No information available.

2. Health Surveillance

No information available.

VI. SUMMARY

ETU causes follicular cell thyroid tumors in rats and liver tumors(?) in mice. It is negative in a wide variety of short-term tests, with only weak positive activity in some tests. ETU is an anti-thyroid agent and probably produces follicular cell tumors in this organ as a result of this nongenotoxic action.

NITRILOTRIACETIC ACID (NTA)

I. CHEMICAL

1. Chemical Structure

Similarity to known carcinogens. None

Reactivity. No information available.

2. Biotransformation and Pharmacokinetics

No detectable metabolism in six mammalian species, including man. Does not alter microsomal enzyme activity. NTA readily absorbed in rodents, not in man; rapidly excreted except for small fraction in bone (Anderson *et al.*, 1982; Budny and Arnold, 1973; Michael and Wakim, 1971).

NTA is absorbed from the gastrointestinal tract by a simple diffusion process. Some 40-60% is absorbed in rodents and excreted only in the urine. When the dietary NTA concentration is about 40 mMolar, the urine must contain NTA that is not complexed with cations, a condition conducive to divalent metal stripping from urinary tract tissues (Anderson *et al.*, 1982; Budny, 1972; Budny and Arnold, 1973; Michael and Wakim, 1971).

3. Biochemical Reactivity

Non-reactive.

II. HOST NON-NEOPLASTIC EFFECTS

1. Relevant Functional Effects in the Host

Rat. Ingestion of high doses of NTA increases the load of zinc entering the renal tubular fluids and such an increased tubular cell resorption of ionic zinc can lead to cellular damage. It is postulated that this is accompanied by hyperplasia and neoplasia (Anderson, 1981; Anderson *et al.*, 1982).

2. Relevant Non-neoplastic Morphologic Effects

Not acutely toxic. NOEL in two-year study 300 mg/kg diet. Levels about 1.5 g/kg diet are nephrotoxic. No other NTA-related lesions found in rats in two-year feeding study (Anderson, 1979a; Anderson and Kanerva, 1978a, 1978b).

Doses of NTA between 1500-5000 ppm are associated with hydropic degeneration in kidney and are observed at six months (Nixon *et al.*, 1972).

No-effect doses of up to 0.5% $Na_3NTA \cdot H_2O$ or H_3NTA in the urothelium have been demonstrated in two 18-24 month studies in rats (NCI, 1977b; Nixon *et al.*, 1972).

III. HOST NEOPLASTIC DETERMINANTS

1. Species and Strains Tested

Mice (Greenblatt and Lijinsky, 1974; NCI, 1977b).
Rats (Goyer *et al.*, 1981; Lijinsky *et al.*, 1973; NCI, 1977b; Nixon *et al.*, 1972).

2. Variety of Histogenetic Tumor Sites in Species Tested

Kidney: rats, mice
Ureter: rat
Bladder: rat

3. Histologic and Biologic Characteristics of Tumors

Kidney: benign and malignant (mice and rats)
Ureter: benign and malignant (rats)
Bladder: benign and malignant (rats)

4. Latent Period in Relation to Dose

Few tumors found before 104 weeks—a few animals dying between 42 and 104 weeks had epithelial tumors of the urogenital tract and/ or kidney.

Table I. Summary of Chronic Exposure Studies with NTA

NTA Form and Dose		Second Treatment	Duration	Urinary Tract Neoplasms		Reference
				Tubular	Transitional Cell	
RAT						
0	Na$_2$NTA in drinking water	—	84 weeks with 20 ml/day on 5 days/week	0/30	0/30	(1)
0.5%		—		1/30	0/30	
0.5%		0.2% NaNO$_2$		2/30	0/30	
0	Na$_3$NTA · H$_2$O in drinking water	—	704 days continuous	5/186	0/186	(2)
0.1%		—		29/183	0/183	
0	Na$_3$NTA · H$_2$O in diet	—	24 months with sacrifices at 19 and 24 months	0/71	0/71	(3)
0.03%		—		0/37	0/37	
0.15%		—		0/31	0/31	
0.50%		—		1/31	0/31	
0.50%	CaNaNTA in diet	—		2/38	0/38	
0	Na$_3$NTA · H$_2$O in diet	—	24 months	0/24	0/24	(4)
0.02%		—		0/48	0/48	
0.2%		—		0/48	1/48*	
2.0%		—		8/48	6/48	

Dose	Compound	Duration			Ref.
0	Na$_3$NTA·H$_2$O in diet	18 months +	0/80	0/80	(4)
0.75%		6 months rest	1/100	4/100	
1.50%			2/100	2/100	
0.75%	H$_3$NTA in diet	18 months +	1/100	2/100	(4)
1.50%		6 months rest	7/100	12/100	
MICE					
0	Na$_2$NTA in drinking water	26 weeks	1/76	1/76	(5)
0.5%		5 ml/day on	1/74	0/74	
0.5%	0.1% NaNO$_2$	5 days/week	0/76	0/76	
0	Na$_3$NTA·H$_2$O in diet	18 months +	0/80	0/80	(4)
0.25%		3 months rest	0/100	0/100	
0.5%			0/100	0/100	
0.75%	H$_3$NTA in diet	18 months +	5/100	0/100	(4)
1.50%		3 months rest	28/100	0/100	

*Papilloma.
(1) Lijinski et al., 1973.
(2) Goyer et al., 1981.
(3) Nixon et al., 1972.
(4) NCI, 1977b.
(5) Greenblatt and Lijinski, 1974.

5. Relationship to Background Tumor Incidence

See Table I. Summary of Chronic Exposure Studies with NTA, Pages 90–91.

6. Qualitative and Quantitative Aspects of Dose-response Relationships

In well-conducted carcinogenicity bioassays.
NTA produces bladder tumors in female rats—15,000 ppm;
NTA produces kidney tumors in male mice—15,000 ppm.

20,000 ppm Na_3NTA produced kidney and bladder tumors in female rats, kidney tumors in male rats, and ureter tumors in both sexes.

IV. SHORT-TERM TESTS

NTA is not a mutagen as attested by its essentially negative response in several assay systems (Foley *et al.*, 1977).

1. Short-Term Tests for Genotoxicity

Mutagenicity
Prokaryotes, mammalian cells, eukaryotes, insects *in vitro* and *in vivo*	neg.	(Kihlman, 1971; Legator, 1971; Lüning, 1970; NCI, 1977b; Pound, 1974; Stine, 1973; Stine and Hardigree, 1972; Zetterberg, 1970)
DNA repair synthesis	neg.	(Williams, 1980c, 1981c)
Sister chromatid exchange	neg.	(Williams *et al.*, 1982)
Chromosomal aberrations	neg.	(Lüning, 1970; Legator, 1970a)
Cell transformation	neg.	(Dunkel, 1979, 1981)

Germ cell effects
Dominant lethal	neg.	(Epstein, 1970; Epstein, *et al.*, 1972; Jorgenson, *et al.*, 1975; Legator, 1970b; Lüning, 1970)
Heritable translocation	neg.	(Jorgenson *et al.*, 1975a)
Host-mediated assay	neg.	(Legator, 1972)

2. Tests for Promotion

> No information available.

V. HUMAN STUDIES

1. Epidemiology

> No information available.

2. Health Surveillance

> No information available.

VI. SUMMARY

> NTA causes urinary tract tumors in rats and mice. It is negative in a variety of short-term tests for genotoxicity but inhibits intercellular communication in V79 cells. Chelation of trace elements leading to the formation of micro-crystalluria may contribute to tumor formation, suggesting a nongenotoxic mechanism.

SACCHARIN

I. CHEMICAL

1. Chemical Structure

> *Similarity to known carcinogens.* Not similar to any known carcinogen.

> *Reactivity.* Very stable with little chemical reactivity. Hydrolysis will occur at high temperatures and extremes of pH (Saccharin Hydrolysis Products, 1982). Two hydrolysis products are o-sulfobenzoic acid and o-sulfamoylbenzoic acid. Sodium saccharin is the salt of a strong organic acid and is in the ionic state in most body fluids.

2. Biotransformation and Pharmacokinetics

> Results of most studies strongly suggest that sodium saccharin is excreted unchanged following oral administration (Ball, 1974; Ball et al., 1977; Byard and Golberg, 1973; Kennedy et al., 1972; Lethco and Wallace, 1975; Minegishi et al., 1972; Pitkin et al., 1971; Renwick and Williams, 1978; Sweatman and Renwick, 1980). Impurities in the saccharin sample or analytical artifacts are the most likely reasons for the reported low levels of biotransformation (Renwick, 1981).

Sodium saccharin is slowly and incompletely absorbed from the gut (60-90% absorbed depending on the species and dose); distributed in the extracellular or total body water; and is rapidly excreted into the urine via glomerular filtration and tubular secretion (Ball *et al.*, 1977; Bekersky *et al.*, 1980; Bourgoignie *et al.*, 1980; Goldstein *et al.*, 1978; Lethco and Wallace, 1975; Renwick and Sweatman, 1979; Sweatman and Renwick, 1980). Sodium saccharin has been shown to cross the placenta (Ball *et al.*, 1977; Mathews *et al.*, 1973). Sodium saccharin has been shown to attain higher tissue levels than would be expected based upon perfusion rates in both fetal and post-neonatal bladder tissue (Ball *et al.*, 1977; Mathews *et al.*, 1973; Sweatman and Renwick, 1980), possibly due to saccharin in the urine adhering to the tissue (Renwick and Sweatman, 1979; Sweatman and Renwick, 1979). All tissues, including the bladder, are rapidly cleared following cessation of exposure.

Studies in man in which sodium saccharin was orally administered have shown that saccharin is well absorbed from the gut (90%) and is excreted unchanged in the urine, mostly within 24 hours after ingestion (Ball *et al.*, 1977; Byard *et al.*, 1974; Sweatman *et al.*, 1981). Following i.v. administration, sodium saccharin has been shown to have a terminal half-life of 70 minutes and to fit a two-compartment open model (Sweatman *et al.*, 1981). In this same study, renal clearance was shown to be high and the dose was quantitatively recovered in the urine. No indication of saturation of renal elimination was found, even at dosages several times higher than the average rate of human consumption.

3. Biochemical Reactivity

Does not form covalent bonds with other compounds. Hydrogen bonding has been reported (Shiffman *et al.*, 1981). Sodium saccharin has been shown to bind to plasma proteins (Anderson, 1979b) but does not bind to DNA of rat liver or bladder (Lutz and Schlatter, 1977).

Sodium saccharin does not undergo electrophilic substitution. It is nucleophilic.

II. HOST NON-NEOPLASTIC EFFECTS

1. Relevant Functional Effects in the Host

The most consistent physiological effect observed is a depression in weight gain (Arnold *et al.*, 1980a; Schoenig and Anderson, 1984; Schoenig *et al.*, 1984; Taylor *et al.*, 1980). At dietary concentrations where tumors have been found ($\geq$ 3%), the effect on body weight loss is considerable, i.e., $\geq$ 10% relative to untreated animals. This effect is more severe in animals with neonatal exposure versus animals whose exposure is started after weaning. The body weight depressions are not due to decrease in nutrient consumption.

Reduction in the litter size of second generation offspring has been observed (Schoenig and Anderson, 1984). This has been observed at dietary concentrations $\geq$ 3%.

Pharmacological effects related to water and mineral balance include increases in water consumption, urine volume and moisture content of feces (Arnold et al., 1980a, 1980b; Demers et al., 1981; Schoenig and Anderson, 1984; Schoenig et al., 1984); increased mineral excretion in the urine (Anderson, 1979a; Arnold et al., 1980a, 1980b; Demers et al., 1981; Schoenig and Anderson, 1984; Schoenig et al., 1984); decreased mineral excretion (except for sodium) in the feces (Anderson, 1979b; Schoenig et al., 1984); decreased osmolality in 24-hour urine samples (Arnold et al., 1980a, 1980b; Demers et al., 1981; Schoenig and Anderson, 1984; Schoenig et al., 1984); and transient changes in urinary pH (Demers et al., 1981; Schoenig et al., 1984). A flocculent urinary precipitate was reported at dietary concentrations of 5% in one two-generation bioassay (Arnold et al., 1980a).

Transient anemia has been observed in weanling rats with neonatal exposure (Schoenig and Anderson, 1984). Clinical chemistry parameters which have been reported as being changed are decreases in serum and urinary glucose (Demers et al., 1981; Thompson and Mayer, 1959).

Both the size and the mass of the cecum are increased in rats fed high dietary concentrations of sodium saccharin (Lawson and Hertzog, 1981; Schoenig et al., 1984). While the size of the bladder in sodium saccharin-treated rats has not been evaluated, the mass of the bladder is significantly increased in rats fed sodium saccharin at dietary concentrations $\geq$ 3% (Schoenig et al., 1984).

The concentration of several minerals (sodium, potassium, magnesium and zinc) has been shown to be significantly increased in the bladder tissue of male rats fed high dietary concentrations of sodium saccharin (Schoenig et al., 1984). There also appears to be an overall cecal retention of some of these minerals (Anderson, 1979b; Schoenig et al., 1984). The fact that the retention of minerals in the bladder is noted in male but not female rats may be a particularly pertinent finding, since bladder tumors are also only observed in male rats.

2. Relevant Non-neoplastic Morphologic Effects

An increase in focal hyperplasia and the occurrence of pleomorphic microvilli have been reported in the bladder tissue of F344 rats fed sodium saccharin at a dietary concentration of 5%. An increase in bladder epithelial DNA synthesis as measured by an increase in uptake of radiolabelled thymidine has been reported in F344 rats (Fukushima and Cohen, 1980; Murasaki and Cohen, 1981).

III. HOST NEOPLASTIC DETERMINANTS

1. Species and Strains Tested

One and two-generation carcinogenicity bioassays have been conducted on sodium saccharin using rats (Arnold *et al.*, 1980a; Bio-research Consultants, 1973; Fitzhugh *et al.*, 1951; Litton Bionetics, 1973; Munro *et al.*, 1975; Schoenig and Anderson, 1984; Taylor, 1980; Tisdel *et al.*, 1974), mice (Bio-research Consultants, 1973; National Institute of Hygienic Sciences Studies, 1973) and hamsters (Althoff *et al.*, 1975) as test animals. A study in which sodium saccharin was fed to monkeys for 6.7 years has also been conducted (Coulston *et al.*, 1975); and another study in which sodium saccharin has been fed to monkeys for approximately 7.5 years is still underway (Sieber and Adamson, 1978).

An increase in bladder tumors has been observed in second generation male Charles River CD rats in three of these studies (Arnold *et al.*, 1980a; Schoenig and Anderson, 1984; Taylor, 1980; Tisdel *et al.*, 1974). In one of the studies an increase in bladder tumors was also observed in first generation male animals (Arnold *et al.*, 1980a). In another study (Schoenig and Anderson, 1984) when exposure to sodium saccharin was initiated at birth, there was a statistically significant increase in the incidence of bladder tumors in the saccharin-treated animals.

2. Variety of Histogenetic Tumor Sites in Species Tested

Urinary bladder epithelium.

3. Histologic and Biologic Characteristics of Tumors

Benign and malignant epithelial tumors. Majority are malignant.

4. Latent Period in Relation to Dose

The mean time-to-tumor appears to be approximately 24 months.

5. Relationship to Background Tumor Incidence

The background tumor incidence for the Charles River CD rat is between 0 and 1%. In the studies where a statistically significant ($p < 0.05$) increase in tumor incidence has been found, the incidence of tumors in saccharin-treated rats has ranged between 18 and 47%.

6. Qualitative and Quantitative Aspects of Dose-response Relationships

In several of the bioassays conducted on sodium saccharin, either only a single dose was evaluated or an increase in tumors was only found at the highest dose level evaluated (5 and 7.5%). In the most recent study (Schoenig and Anderson, 1984) which tested saccharin in the male rat at dosage levels of 1.00, 3.00, 4.00, 5.00, 6.25, and 7.50% in diet; the tumor response decreased rapidly with reductions in dose level. In the initial review of the pathology, a statistically significant incidence of bladder tumors was noted at dose levels of 3% and above. At the 3% dose level, signficance was only obtained when malignant and benign tumors were combined. In a subsequent independent and blind review of the pathology by Dr. Robert Squire, a significant incidence of bladder tumors was found only at dose levels of 4% and above.

IV. SHORT-TERM TESTS

1. Short-Term Tests for Genotoxicity

Mutagenicity[2]

Bacteria	(Batzinger et al., 1977; Litton Bionetics, 1978; McCann, 1977; Pool, 1978; Stoltz et al., 1977)
Yeast	(McCann, 1977; Moore and Schmick, 1979; Simmon, 1979a)
Mammalian cells	(Clive et al., 1979; McCann, 1977)

---

[2]Occasionally, weak activity has been reported in the bacterial cell genetic assays, and some activity has been reported for sodium saccharin in most, but not all, of the mammalian cell genetic assays. However, in all studies where activity has been reported, very high and often toxic dose levels were used. In addition, usually no dose-response was obtained, or the criteria for identifying positive activity was modified downward. Even deliberate attempts by independent investigators to reproduce reported positive findings for sodium saccharin in several of these assays resulted in highly inconsistent results, and the observation of activity similar to that reported for sodium saccharin with three vitamins which are normal constituents of many foods, i.e., ascorbic acid, pantothenic acid and ergocalciferol.

Chromosomal aberrations	(Abe and Sasaki, 1977; Ishidate and Odashima, 1977; Kristofferson, 1972; Masubuchi et al., 1978; McCann, 1977; Newell and Maxwell, 1972; Ochi and Tonomura, 1978; Stone et al., 1969)
Sister chromatid exchange	(Abe and Sasaki, 1977; Saxholm et al., 1979; Wolff and Rodin, 1978)

Nine functional analogs of sodium saccharin have been evaluated in the *Salmonella* mutagenicity assay (four tester strains) and cell transformation assay (baby hamster kidney cells) and were found to be negative in both assays (Ashby et al., 1978).

2. Tests for Promotion

Saccharin has been evaluated for tumor-promoting activity in several bioassays in which potent bladder carcinogens have been used as initiators (Cohen et al., 1979b; Fukushima et al., 1981; Green et al., 1980; Hicks and Chowaniec, 1977). In several of these bioassays positive responses have been obtained in male and female rats at sodium saccharin dietary concentrations of 5% (Cohen et al., 1979b; Connolly et al., 1978; Fukushima et al., 1981; Hicks and Chowaniec, 1977). The essential amino acid, tryptophan, was also shown to have promoting activity in two of these initiation/ promotion bioassays (Cohen et al., 1979b; Fukushima et al., 1981). The histogenetic type of tumors observed have been similar to those found in the classical carcinogenicity bioassay, i.e., transitional cell papillomas and carcinomas.

No activity has been observed with sodium saccharin in four separate transformation assays using mammalian cells from three different species as target organisms (Ashby et al., 1978; McCann, 1977; Mondal et al., 1978; Sivak, 1979).

V. HUMAN STUDIES

1. Epidemiology

Temporal trend studies (Armstrong and Doll, 1974; Burbank and Fraumeni, 1970), cohort studies in diabetics (Armstrong et al., 1976; Kessler, 1970), and case-control studies (Chapman et al.,

1979; Connolly *et al.*, 1978; Hoover, 1980; Hoover and Strasser, 1980; Howe *et al.*, 1980; Kessler, 1976, 1978; Miller and Howe, 1977; Miller *et al.*, 1978; Morgan and Jain, 1974; Morrison and Buring, 1980; Newell *et al.*, 1978; Simon *et al.*, 1975; Wynder and Goldsmith, 1977; Wynder and Stellman, 1980) have been conducted in order to evaluate the association between bladder cancer and the use of sodium saccharin. No reproducible positive findings have been noted in any of these studies, including one of the largest case-control studies ever conducted (Hoover and Strasser, 1980). While some authors of the case-control studies have raised questions regarding some subgroups within their studies (Hoover and Strasser, 1980; Miller and Howe, 1977; Morrison and Buring, 1980; Wynder and Stellman, 1980), none of the studies conducted to date have resulted in a statistically significant association when all cases were compared to all controls.

2. Health Surveillance

No information available.

VI. SUMMARY

Saccharin was associated with bladder tumors in male Charles River CD rats but not in other rat strains or in mice and hamsters. The compound was nongenotoxic in short-term tests, except for very high doses, when in some cases a very weak positive reaction was found. It has been shown to be a promoter in bladder carcinogenesis in the rat and seems to cause a retention of minerals in the bladder, especially in male rats.

Saccharin is nongenotoxic, and in the rat shows promoter activity in bladder carcinogenesis. The precise mechanism of action for carcinogenicity is unclear.

2,3,7,8-TETRACHLORODIBENZO-p-DIOXIN (TCDD)

I. CHEMICAL

1. Chemical Structure

Similarity to known carcinogens. No structural analogies on which to base an expectation of carcinogenicity.

Reactivity. Stable in environmental media.

2. Biotransformation and Pharmacokinetics

> Very slowly metabolized; TCDD is metabolized to more than one metabolite, some of which bind preferentially to protein (Gunther *et al.*, 1979).

3. Biochemical Reactivity

> *Electrophilic substitution.* Very low binding-6 and 12 pmol/mol nucleotide residue 99.9% of (^{3}H) TCDD dose was extractable. Binding to DNA is equivalent to one molecule TCDD per DNA equivalent to 35 cells (Poland and Glover, 1979).

II. HOST NON-NEOPLASTIC EFFECTS

1. Relevant Functional Effects in the Host

> *Physiological.* Suppression of cell mediated immunity.
> *Biochemical.* Potent inducer of hepatic and renal microsomal enzymes (Dees *et al.*, 1982; Poland and Kende, 1976). Marked increase in cellular smooth endoplasmic reticulum in liver and kidney.

2. Relevant Non-neoplastic Morphologic Effects

> *Nature/degree.* Hepatic cell necrosis, thymic atrophy, depletion of lymphoid organs. The degree of hepatic involvement appears to be dose-dependent and severity of change produced varies among species (Harris *et al.*, 1973; Schwetz *et al.*, 1973; Vos *et al.*, 1973).

III. HOST NEOPLASTIC DETERMINANTS

1. Species and Strains Tested
    Rats, mice (Kociba *et al.*, 1978; NCI, 1980a, 1980b; Toth *et al.*, 1979; Van Miller *et al.*, 1977).

2. Variety of Histogenetic Tumor Sites in Species Tested
    Rat (Sprague-Dawley) (Kociba *et al.*, 1978).

μg/kg bw	*Male* 0	%	0.01	%	0.1	%
Squamous cell carcinoma of						
palatum + turbinates	0/85	(0)	0/50	(0)	4/50	(8)
lung	0/85	(0)	1/50	(2)	3/50	(8)
total squamous carcinoma	0/85	(0)	0/50	(2)	7/50	(14)
liver hepatocellular carcinoma	2/85	(2)	0/50	(0)	1/50	(2)

μg/kg bw	0	%	0.01	%	0.1	%
Female						
Squamous cell carcinoma of palatum + turbinates	0/86	(0)	1/50	(2)	4/49	(8)
lung	0/86	(0)	0/50	(0)	7/49	(14)
total squamous carcinoma	0/86	(0)	1/50	(2)	11/49	(22)
liver hepatocellular carcinoma	0/86	(0)	2/50	(4)	11/49	(22)

Rat (Osborne Mendel). Increased incidence thyroid tumors in males. Lung: 2,10,16 and 22% in 0,0.1,0.05 and 0.06 μg/kg bw. Increased hepatocellular carcinoma incidence only in highest dose group female.

Mice (B6C3F$_1$). Increased liver carcinoma incidence at highest dose in male as well as female.

Doses used.

> male   0, 0.01, 0.05, 0.5 μg/kg bw
> female   0, 0.04, 0.2, 2 μg/kg bw (NCI, 1980a, 1980b)

Increased liver tumor incidence at highest dose and next lower dose. Inconclusive study (Van Miller, 1977).
Increased liver tumor incidence at highest dose and next lower dose. Inconclusive study (Toth *et al.*, 1979).

3. Histologic and Biologic Characteristics of Tumors

> Mainly malignant in 1 mg/kg/day.
> Mainly benign at 0.01 mg/kg/day.

4. Latent Period in Relation to Dose

> 0.1 μg/kg/day for two years
> 0.001 and 0.01 μg/kg/day produced no tumor increase in rats.

5. Relationship to Background Tumor Incidence

> Approximately 20% benign tumors including neoplastic nodules.

6. Qualitative and Quantitative Aspects of Dose-response Relationships

> An apparent NOEL for all tumor types at 0.001 μg/kg/day.

IV. SHORT-TERM TESTS

1. Short-Term Tests for Genotoxicity

Mutagenicity	pos.	Results reported by some authors: cytotoxicity cannot be excluded as a cause (Hussain *et al.*, 1972; Seiler, 1973)
	neg.	Results by other authors: (Gilbert et al., 1980; Geiger and Neal, 1981; Nebert *et al.*, 1976; Wassom *et al.*, 1978)
Yeast	pos.	(Bronzetti *et al.*, 1980)
Drosophila	neg.	(Mason *et al.*, 1981)
Chromosomal aberrations	neg.	(Green and Moreland, 1975; Sbrana *et al.*, 1980)
DNA repair synthesis	neg.	(Sbrana *et al.*, 1980)
Germ cell effects	neg.	(Khera and Ruddick, 1973)

2. Tests for Promotion

Potent promoting agent for hepatocarcinogenesis (Pitot *et al.*, 1980). No initiating nor promoting activity in skin (Berry *et al.*, 1978; DiGiovanni *et al.*, 1977; NCI, 1980b).

Anti-initiating activities (Berry *et al.*, 1979; Cohen *et al.*, 1979a; DiGiovanni, 1977).

V. HUMAN STUDIES

1. Epidemiology

Acute and subchronic exposure have demonstrated that humans are far less susceptible than laboratory animals (IARC, 1977). The data also indicate the presence of chloracne as a marker preceding other potential health effects.

No reports are available of human exposure only to TCDD. Men exposed to TCDD during the manufacture or use of 2,4,5-trichlorophenol and/or 2,4,5-T production (IARC, 1982).

2. Health Surveillance

No information available.

VI. SUMMARY

TCDD caused a variety of tumors in rats and mice. In genotoxicity tests, TCDD was negative except in some studies where cytotoxic doses were used. It has strong promoting activity in liver carcinogenesis but none in skin carcinogenicity.

TCDD has shown to be a very potent nongenotoxic carcinogen; the mechanism of action has yet to be elucidated.

TETRACHLOROETHYLENE
(PERCHLOROETHYLENE, ETHYLENETETRACHLORIDE)

I. CHEMICAL

1. Chemical Structure

Similarity to known carcinogens. Trichloroethylene.

Reactivity. No information available.

2. Biotransformation and Pharmacokinetics

Tetrachloroethylene is metabolized to trichloroacetylchloride, which is further metabolized to trichloroacetic acid and trichloroethanol (Daniel, 1963; Ogata *et al.*, 1971; Yllner, 1961).

Tetrachloroethylene is only partly (2-20%) metabolized (IARC, 1979c). Half-times vary from 7-65 hours (Pegg *et al.*, 1979; Stewart *et al.*, 1974). Metabolism can be stimulated by drug metabolism enzymes (Moslen *et al.*, 1977).

In humans tetrachloroethylene is very slowly metabolized (Ikeda, 1977; Ikeda and Imamura, 1973; Münzer and Heder, 1972; Ogata *et al.*, 1971).

3. Biochemical Reactivity

No DNA binding (Schumann and Watanabe, 1979; Schumann *et al.*, 1980).

Since metabolism does occur, and epoxides may be formed, some reactive binding cannot be excluded. No information on this particular phenomenon is available.

II. HOST NON-NEOPLASTIC EFFECTS

1. Relevant Functional Effects in the Host

LD50 oral—6.4–13 g/kg bw
LD50 i.p.—3.5–7 g/kg bw
LC50—5200 ppm

Hepatotoxic, nephrotoxic, narcotic, embryotoxic, not teratogenic (Parker *et al.*, 1978; Schwetz *et al.*, 1975).

2. Relevant Non-neoplastic Morphologic Effects

Liver and kidney degeneration, liver cirrhosis

III. HOST NEOPLASTIC DETERMINANTS

1. Species and Strains Tested

Only found to lead to increased tumor incidence in $B6C3F_1$ mice (Weisburger, 1977).

Mouse skin	neg.	(van Duuren *et al.*, 1979)
Mouse i.p.	neg.	(Theiss *et al.*, 1977)
Rat oral	neg.	(Weisburger, 1977)
Rat inhalation	neg.	(Rampy *et al.*, 1977)

Increased liver tumor incidence	0	Medium Dose	High Dose
Male	4/47	32/49	27/48
Female	2/40	19/48	19/48

2. Variety of Histogenetic Tumor Sites in Species Tested

Only liver was affected.

3. Histologic and Biologic Characteristics of Tumors

Hepatocellular carcinoma.

4. Latent Period in Relation to Dose

No information available.

5. Relationship to Background Tumor Incidence

See 3: mice had a low background incidence for liver carcinoma.

6. Qualitative and Quantitative Aspects of Dose-response Relationships

See 1 above.

IV. SHORT-TERM TESTS

1. Short-Term Tests for Genotoxicity

Mutagenicity

Bacteria	neg.	(Bartsch *et al.*, 1979; Greim *et al.*, 1977a, 1977b; IARC, 1979b, 1979c)
	marginal	(Callen *et al.*, 1980)
Chromosomal aberrations	neg.	(IARC, 1979c; Ikeda *et al.*, 1980)
Cell transformation	pos.	(Price *et al.*, 1978)

2. Tests for Promotion

No information available.

V. HUMAN STUDIES

1. Epidemiology

No adequate epidemiological studies are available. In a mortality study comprising death certificates of former laundry workers a slight excess in deaths over expected was observed. However, exposure to other solvents must have occurred as well (IARC, 1982).

2. Health Surveillance

No information available.

VI. SUMMARY

Tetrachloroethylene caused only liver tumors in mice. *In vitro* short-term tests for genotoxicity were negative and binding to DNA does not occur. The compound is hepatotoxic and causes cirrhosis.

Tetrachloroethylene is a nongenotoxic carcinogen which induces only liver tumors in mice. This effect is probably related to its hepatotoxicity.

X. References

Abe, S. and Sasaki, M. (1977). Chromosome aberrations and sister chromatid exchanges in Chinese hamster cells exposed to various chemicals. *Mutat. Res., 48*, 337-354.

Abraham, R. and Hendy, R.J. (1970). Irreversible lysosomal damage induced by chloroquine in the retina of pigmented and albino rats. *Exp. Mol. Pathol., 12*, 185-200.

Agnew, L.R.C. and Gardner, W.U. (1952). Spontaneous hepatomas - effect of estrogen and androgen on the occurrence of these tumors in C_3H mice. *Cancer Res., 12*, 757-761.

Agthe, C., Garcia, H., Shubik, P., Tomatis, L. and Wenyon, E. (1970). Study of the potential carcinogenicity of DDT in Syrian golden hamsters. *Proc. Soc. Exp. Biol. Med., 134*, 113-116.

Ahmed, F.E., Lewis, N.J. and Hart, R.W. (1977a). Pesticide induced ouabain resistant mutants in Chinese hamster V79 cells. *Chem.-Biol. Interact., 19*, 369-374.

Ahmed, F.E., Hart, R.W. and Lewis, N.J. (1977b). Pesticide induced DNA damage and its repair in cultured human cells. *Mutat. Res., 42*, 161-174.

Alexander, P. (1982). Prostaglandins and cancer. *Nature, 295*, 188-189.

Althoff, J., Cardesa, A., Pour, P. and Shubik, P. (1975). A chronic study of artificial sweeteners in Syrian Golden Hamsters. *Cancer Lett., 1*, 121-124.

Alvarez, A.P. (1977). Stimulatory effects of polychlorinatedbiphenyls (PCB) on cyto-chromes P-450 and P-448 mediated microsomal oxidations, In *Microsomes and Drug Oxidations,*(V. Ullrich, A. Hildebrandt, I. Roots, R. W. Estabrook and A. H. Conney, eds.), p. 476, Pergamon Press, New York.

Ames, B.N., McCann, J. and Yamasaki, E. (1975). Methods for detecting carcinogens with the *Salmonella*/mammalian microsome mutagenicity test. *Mutat. Res., 31*, 347-364.

Amiel, J.L. (1960). Essai négatif d'induction de leucémies chez les souris par la benzène. *Rev. Fr. Etud. Clin. Biol., 5*, 198-199.

Amkraut, A. and Solomon, G.F. (1972). Stress and murine sarcoma virus (Moloney)-induced tumors. *Cancer Res., 32*, 1428-1433.

Anderson, K.V., Coyle, F.P., and O'Steen, W.K. (1972). Retinal degeneration produced by low-intensity colored light. *Exp. Neurol., 35*, 233-238.

Anderson, R.L. (1979a). Discontinuities in dose-response curves from toxicological tests. Oral presentation at the Soap and Detergent Association Annual Meeting in *Soap Cosmetics Chemical Specialties*, p. 36, Boca Raton.

Anderson, R.L. (1979b). Response of male rats to sodium saccharin ingestion: urine composition and mineral balance. *Food Cosmet. Toxicol., 17*, 195-200.

Anderson, R.L. (1981). The role of zinc in nitrilotriacetate (NTA)-associated renal tubular cell toxicity. *Food Cosmet. Toxicol., 19*, 639.

Anderson, R.L., Alden, C.L. and Merski, J.A. (1982). The effects of nitrilotriacetate on cation disposition and urinary tract toxicity. *Food Cosmet. Toxicol., 20*, 105-122.

Anderson, R.L. and Kanerva, R.L. (1978a). Effect of nitrilotriacetate (NTA) on cation balance in the rat. *Food Cosmet. Toxicol. 16*, 563.

Anderson, R.L. and Kanerva, R.L. (1978b). Hypercalcinuria and crystalluria during ingestion of dietary nitrilotriacetate. *Food Cosmet. Toxicol., 16*, 569.

Andrews, L.S., Lee, E.W., Witmer, C.M., Kocsis, J.J., and Snyder, R. (1977). Effects of toluene on the metabolism, disposition and the hemopoietic toxicity of [^{3}H]- benzene. *Biochem. Pharmacol., 26*, 293-300.

Anisman, H., Suissa, A. and Sklar, L.S. (1980). Escape deficits induced by uncontrollable stress: antagonism by dopamine and norepinephrine agonists. *Behav. Neural. Biol., 28*, 34-37.

Anon. (1981). Unpublished studies cited by Japan Medical Gazette, January 20, 1981.

Arfellini, G., Grilli, S. and Prodi, G.(1978). *In vivo* DNA repair after N-methyl-N-nitrosourea administration to rats of different ages. *Z. Krebforsch Klin. Onkol., 91*, 157-164.

Armstrong, B. and Doll, R. (1974). Bladder cancer mortality in England and Wales in relation to cigarette smoking and saccharin consumption. *Br. J. Prev. Soc. Med., 28*, 233-240.

Armstrong, B., Lea, A.J., Adelstein, A.M., Donovan, J.W., White G.C. and Ruttle, S. (1976). Cancer mortality and saccharin consumption in diabetics. *Br. J. Prev. Soc. Med., 39*, 151-157.

Arnold, D.W., Kennedy, G.L., Keplinger, M.L., Calandra, J.C. and Calo, C.J. (1977). Dominant lethal studies with technical chlordane, HCS-3260, and heptachlor: heptachlor epoxide. *J. Toxicol. Environ. Health, 2*, 547.

Arnold, D.L., Fox, J.G., Thibert, P. and Grice, H.C. (1978). Toxicology studies I. Support personnel. *Food Cosmet. Toxicol., 16*, 479-484.

Arnold, D.L. and Grice, H.C. (1979). The use of the Syrian hamster in toxicology studies with emphasis on carcinogenesis bioassay. *Prog. Exp.Tumor Res., 24*, 222-234.

Arnold, D.L., Moodie, C.A., Grice, H.C., Charbonneau, S.M., Stavric, B., Collins, B.T., McGuire, P.F., Zawidzka, Z.Z. and Munro, I.C. (1980a). Long-term toxicity of ortho-toluenesulfonamide and sodium saccharin in the rat. *Toxicol. Appl. Pharmacol., 52*, 113-152.

Arnold. D.L., Stavric, B., McGuire, P.F. and Munro, I.C. (1980b). The effect of sodium saccharin on several urinary parameters in the rat. Society of Toxicology meeting, Washington, Paper No. 228.

Arnold, D.L., Bickis, M., Nera, E., McGuire, P. and Munro, I.C. (1982). Assessing the reversibility of thyroid lesions that result from feeding ETU. Society of Toxicology Annual Meeting, abstract.

Arnold, D.L., Krewski, D., Junkins, D.B., McGuire, P.F., Moodie, C.A. and Munro, I.C. (1983). Reversibility of ethylenethiourea induced thyroid lesions. *Toxicol. Appl. Pharmacol., 69*, 264-273.

Asher, I.M. and Zervos, C.(eds.) (1978). *Structural Correlates of Carcinogenesis and Mutagenesis: A Guide to Testing Priorities?* Proceedings of the Second Food and Drug Administration Office of Science Summer Symposium, Rockville, Maryland.

Ashby, J., Styles, J.A., Anderson, D. and Paton, D. (1978). Saccharin an epigenetic carcinogen/mutagen? *Food Cosmet. Toxicol., 16*, 95-103.

Ashwood-Smith, M.J., Trevion, J. and Ring, R. (1972). Mutagenicity of dichlorvos. *Nature (London), 240*, 418-419.

Astrin, S.M. and Rothberg, P.G. (1983). Oncogenes and cancer. *Cancer Invest.*, *1*, 355-364.

Austin, G. and Moyer, G. (1979). Hepatic RNA synthesis in rats treated with ethylene-thiourea. *Res. Commun. Chem. Pathol. Pharmacol.*, *23*, 639-642.

Baldwin, R.W. (1973). Immunological aspects of chemical carcinogenesis. *Adv. Cancer Res. 18*, 1-75.

Ball, L.M. (1974). The metabolic fate of $[14^C]$ saccharin in rats chronically fed on saccharin compounds. 550th meeting, *Biochemical Society Transactions, 2*, Englefield Green, London.

Ball, L.M., Renwick, A.G., Williams, R.T. (1977). The fate of $[^{14}C]$ saccharin in man, rat and rabbit and of 2-sulphamoyl $[^{14}C]$ benzoic acid in the rat. *Xenobiotica, 7*, 189-203.

Barnard, S.D. (1979). Effects of the hypocholesterolemic agents probucol and clofibrate on hepatic ultrastructure. *Toxicol. Appl. Pharmacol., 48*, A98.

Barnard, S.D., Mollelo, J.A., Caldwell, W.J. and LeBeau, J.E.(1980) Comparative ultrastructural study of rat hepatocytes after treatment with hypolipidemic agents probucol, clofibrate and fenofibrate. *J. Toxicol. Environ. Health, 6*, 547.

Barrows, L.R., and Shank, R.C. (1981). Aberrant methylation of liver DNA in rats during hepatotoxicity. *Toxicol. Appl. Pharmacol., 60*, 334-345.

Bartsch, H., Malaveille, C., Barbin, A. and Plunche, G.(1979).Mutagenic and alkylating metabolites of halo-ethylenes, chlorobutadienes and dichlorobutenes produced by rodent or human liver tissues. *Arch. Toxicol., 41*, 249-277.

Bartsch, H., Malaveille, C., Camus, A., Martel-Plance, G., Brun, G. Hautefeuille, A., Sabadie, N., Barbin, A., Kuroki, T., Drevon, C., Piccoli, C. and Montesano, R. (1980). Bacterial and mammalian mutagenicity tests: validation and comparative studies on 180 chemicals. In *Molecular and Cellular Aspects of Carcinogen Screening Tests* (R. Montesano, H. Bartsch and L. Tomatis, eds.), pp.179-242, International Agency for Research on Cancer, Lyon.

Bartsch, H., Tomatis, L. and Malaveille, C. (1982). Mutagenicity and carcinogenicity of environmental chemicals. *Reg. Toxicol. Pharmacol., 2*, 94-105.

Baty, J.D. (1979). Species, strain and sex differences in metabolism. In *Foreign Compounds Metabolism in Mammals* (D.E. Hathway, ed.) Volume 5, pp. 159-189, Chemical Society of London.

Baty, J.D. (1981). Species, strain and sex differences in metabolism. In *Foreign Compounds Metabolism in Mammals* (D.E. Hathway, ed.) Volume 6, pp. 133-159, Chemical Society of London.

Batzinger, R.P., Ou, S.Y.L., and Bueding, E. (1977). Saccharin and other sweeteners: mutagenic properties. *Science, 198*, 944-946.

Bekersky, I., Poynor, W.J. and Colburn, W.A. (1980). Pharmacokinetics of saccharin in the rat. *Drug Metab. Dispos., 8*, 64.

Beland, F.A., Beranek, D.T., Dooley, K.L., Heflich, R.H. and Kadlubar, F.F. (1983). Arylamine-DNA adducts *in vitro* and *in vivo*: their role in bacterial mutagenesis and urinary bladder carcinogenesis. *Environ. Health Perspect., 49*, 125-134.

Bellhorn, R.W. (1980). Lighting in the animal environment. *Lab. Anim. Sci., 30*, 440-450.

Berenblum, I. (1929). Tumor formation following freezing with carbon dioxide snow. *Br. J. Exp. Pathol., 10*, 179.

Berenblum, I. (1944). Irritation and carcinogenesis. *Arch. Pathol., 38*, 233.

Berenblum, I. and Shubik, P. (1947a). The role of croton oil applications, associated with a single painting of a carcinogen, in tumour induction of the mouse's skin. *Br. J. Cancer, 1*, 379-383.

Berenblum, I. and Shubik, P. (1947b). A new quantitative approach to the study of the stages of chemical carcinogenesis in the mouse's skin. *Br. J. Cancer, 1*, 384-386.

Berenblum, I. and Shubik, P. (1949). The persistence of latent tumour cells induced in the mouse's skin by a single application of 9,10-dimethyl-1,2-benzanthracene. *Br. J. Cancer, 3*, 384-386.

Berqquist, A., Kullander, S., and Thorells, J. (1981). A study of estrogen and progesterone cytosol receptor concentrations in benign and malignant ovarian tumors and a review of malignant ovarian tumors treated with medroxyprogesterone acetate. *Acta Obstet. Gynecol. Scand. Suppl., 101*, 75-81.

Berry, D.L., DiGiovanni, J., Juchau, M.R., Bracken, W.M., Gleason, G.L. and Slaga, T.J. (1978). Lack of tumor-promoting ability of certain environmental chemicals in a two-stage mouse skin tumorigenesis assay. *Res. Commun. Chem. Pathol. Pharmacol., 20*, 101-108.

Berry, D.L., Slaga, T.J., DiGiovanni, J. and Juchau, M.R. (1979). Studies with chlorinated dibenzo-p-dioxins, polybrominated biphenyls and polychlorinated biphenyls in a two-stage system of mouse skin tumorigenesis: Potent anti-carcinogenic effects. *Ann. N.Y. Acad. Sci., 320*, 405-414.

Bielschowsky, F. (1949). The role of thyroxine deficiency in the formation of experimental tumors of the thyroid. *Br. J. Cancer, 3*, 547.

Bickis, M. and Krewski, D. (1984). Statistical design and analysis of the long-term carcinogenicity bioassay. In *Toxicological Risk Assessment* (D. Clayson, D. Krewski and I. Munro, eds.), CRC Press, Boca Raton, In Press.

Bier, O.G., DaSilva, W.D., Götze, D. and Mota, I. (1981). *Fundamentals of Immunology*, Springer-Verlag, New York.

Bio-Research Consultants, Inc. (1973). Studies on saccharin and cyclamate - final report. Contract NIH-NCI-E-68-1311, May 31, 1973.

Bischoff, F. and Bryson, G. (1964). Carcinogenesis through solid state surfaces. *Prog. Exp. Tumor Res., 5*, 85-97.

Blackwell-Smith, R., Finnegan, J., Larson, P., Sahyoun, P., Dreyfuss, M. and Haag, H. (1953). Toxicological studies on zinc and disodium ethylene bis-dithiocarbamates. *J. Pharmacol. Exp. Ther., 109*, 159-166.

Blair, D.G., Oskarsson, M. and Wood, T.G. (1981). Activation of the transforming potential of a normal cell sequence: a molecular model for oncogenesis. *Science, 212*, 941-943.

Boorman, G.A. and Hollander, D.F. (1974). High incidence of spontaneous urinary bladder and ureter tumors in the brown Norway rat. *J. Natl. Cancer Inst., 52*, 1685-1689.

Booth, J., Boyland, E., and Cooling, C. (1967). The respiration of human liver tissue. *Biochem. Pharmacol.,16*, 721-724.

Booth, S.C., Bosenber, H., Garner, R.C., Hertzog, P.J. and Morpoth, K. (1981). The activation of aflatoxin B_1 in liver slices and in bacterial mutagenicity assays using livers from different species including man. *Carcinogenesis, 2*, 1063-1068.

Bourgoignie, J.J., Hwang, K.H., Pennel, J.P. and Bricker, N.S. (1980). Renal excretion of saccharin. *Am. J. Physiol., 238*, F10-F15.

Boutwell, R.K. (1974). The function and mechanism of promoters in carcinogenesis. *CRC Crit. Rev. Toxicol., 2*, 419-443.

Boveri, T. (1929). *The Origin of Malignant Tumors*. Williams and Wilkins, Maryland.

Bowman, M.C. (1969). *Carcinogens and Related Substances*, pp. 23-58, M. Dekker, New York.

Boylan, J.J. Egle, J.L. and Guzelian, P.S. (1978). Cholestyramine: use as a new therapeutic approach for chlordecone (Kepone) poisoning. *Science, 199*, 893.

Brand, K.G. (1975). Foreign body induced sarcomas. In *Cancer, Comprehensive Treatise* (F.F. Becker, ed.), Vol 1. pp. 485-511, Plenum Press, New York.

Brandt, W.N., Flamm, W.G. and Bernheim, N.J. (1972). The value of hydroxyurea in assessing repair synthesis of DNA in HeLa cells. *Chem.-Biol. Interact., 5*, 327-339.

Bridges, B.A., MacGregor, D., Zeiger, E., Bonin, A., Dean, B.J., Lorenzo, G., Garner, R.C., Gatehouse, D. and Hubbard, S. (1981). Summary report on the performance of bacterial mutation assays. *Prog. Mutat. Res., 1*, 49-67.

Broder, S., Muul, L. and Waldmann, T.A. (1978). Suppressor cells in neoplastic disease. *J. Natl. Cancer Inst., 61*, 5-11.

Brodie, B.B., Reid, W.D., Cho, A.K., Spies, G., Krishna, G. and Gillette, J.R. (1971). Possible mechanism of liver necrosis caused by aromatic organic compounds, *Proc. Natl. Acad. Sci .U.S.A., 68*, 160.

Bro-Jorgensen, K., Guttler, F., Jorgensen, P.N., and Volkert, M. (1975). T-lymphocyte function as the principal target of lymphocytic choriomeningitis virus-induced immuno-suppression. *Infect. Immunol., 11*, 622-629.

Bronzetti, G., Lee, I., Zeiger, E., Malling, H. and Suzuki (1980). Genetic effects of TCDD *in vitro* and *in vivo* using D_7 strain of *Saccharomyces cerevisiae. Mutat. Res., 74*, 206-207 (abstract).

Brookes, P., and Preston, R.J. (1981). Summary report on the performance of *in vitro* mammalian assays. *Prog. Mutat. Res., 1*, 77-85.

Brown, K.G. and Hoel, D.G. (1983). Modeling time-to tumor data: analysis of the ED_{01} study. *Fund. Appl. Toxicol., 3*, 458-469.

Brown, C. and Koziol, J. (1983). Statistical aspects of the estimation of human risk from suspected environmental carcinogens. *Soc. Ind. Appl. Math. Rev., 25*, 151-181.

Brown, M.M., Wassom, J.S., Malling H.V., Shelby, M.D. and Von Halle, G.S. (1979). Literature survey of bacterial, fungal and *Drosophila* assay systems used in the evaluation of selected chemical compounds of mutagenic activity. *J. Natl. Cancer Inst., 62,* 841-871.

Brunda, M.J., Herberman, R.B. and Holden, H.T. (1980). Inhibition of murine natural killer cell activity by prostaglandins. *J. Immunol., 124,* 2682-2687.

Budny, J.A. (1972). Metabolism and blood pressure effects of disodium nitrilotriacetate (Na_3NTA) in dogs. *Toxicol. Appl. Pharmacol., 22,* 655.

Budny, J.A. and Arnold, J.D. (1973). Nitrilotriacetate (NTA); human metabolism and its importance in the total safety evaluation program. *Toxicol. Appl. Pharmacol., 25,* 48.

Burbank, F. and Fraumeni, J.F., Jr. (1970). Synthetic sweetener consumption and bladder cancer trends in the United States. *Nature, 227,* 296-297.

Burchfield, H.P.,Storrs, E.E. and Green, R.E. (1977). Role of analytical chemistry in carcinogenesis studies. In *Advances in Modern Toxicology* (H.F. Kraybill and M.A. Mehlman, eds.), pp. 108-113, Hemisphere, Washington.

Burdette, W.J. and Strong, L.C. (1941). Comparison of methyl salicylate and benzene as solvents for methylcholanthrene. *Cancer Res., 1,* 939-941.

Burke, M.D. and Upshall, D.G. (1976). Species and phenobarbitone-induced differences in the kinetic constants of liver microsomal harmine O-demethylation. *Xenobiotica, 6,* 321.

Burnet, F.M. (1970). The concept of immunological surveillance. *Prog. Exp. Tumor Res., 13,* 1-27.

Byard, J.L. and Golberg, L. (1973). The metabolism of saccharin in laboratory animals. *Food Cosmet. Toxicol., 11,* 391-402.

Byard, J.L., McChesney, E.W., Golberg, L. and Coulston, F. (1974). Excretion and metabolism of saccharin in man. II. Studies with [^{14}C] labelled and unlabelled saccharin. *Food Cosmet. Toxicol., 12,* 175.

Cabral, J.R.P., Hall, R.K., Rosse, L., Bronczyk, S. and Shubik, P. (1980). Comparative chronic toxicity of DDT in rats and hamsters. Abstracts, Society of Toxicology, p. A137.

Caldwell, J. (1981). The current status of attempts to predict species differences in drug metabolism. *Drug Metab. Rev., 12,* 221.

Caldwell, J., Notarianni, L.J., Smith, R.L., Fafunsu, M.A., French, M.R., Dawson, P. and Bossir, O. (1979). Non human primate species as metabolic models for the human situation: comparative studies on meperidine metabolism. *Toxicol. Appl. Pharmacol., 48,* 273-278.

Callen, D.F., Wolf, C.R., and Philpot, R.M. (1980). Cytochrome P-450 mediated genetic activity and cytotoxicity of seven halogenated aliphatic hydrocarbons in *Saccharomyces cerevisiae. Mutat. Res.,* 77, 55-63.

Cameron, R.G., Imaida, K., Tsuda, M. and Ito, N. (1982). Promotive effects of steroids and bile acids on hepatocarcinogenesis initiated by diethylnitrosamine. *Cancer Res., 42,* 2426-2428.

Cardinali, D.P. (1981). Melatonin, a mammalian pineal hormone. *Endocr. Rev., 2*, 327-346.

Carroll, K.K. (1980). Lipids and carcinogenesis. *J. Environ. Pathol. Toxicol., 3*, 253-271.

Casarett, L.J. and Doull, J. (eds.) (1975). *Toxicology, The Basic Science of Poisons.* MacMillan Publishing, New York.

Chapman, J.W., Connolly, J.G. and Rosenbaum, L. (1979). Bladder cancer: a case-control study. Occupation and artificial sweeteners. *Toronto Bladder Cancer Symposium,* November, 1979.

Chedid, A. and Nair, V. (1971). Diurnal rhythm in endoplasmic reticulum of rat liver: electron microscopic study. *Science, 175,* 176-179.

Chisnell, C.F., Sik, R.H., Gladen, B.C. and Feldman, D.B. (1981). The effects of different types of fluorescent lighting on reproduction and tumor development in the C_3H mouse. *Photochem. Photobiol., 34,* 617-621.

Chu, E.H.Y. and Malling, H.V. (1968). Mammalian cell genetics II. Chemical induction of specific locus mutations in Chinese hamster cells *in vitro. Proc. Natl. Acad. Sci. U.S.A., 61,* 1306-1312.

Clark, E.A., Russell, P.H., Egghart, M. and Horton, M.A. (1979). Characteristic and genetic control of NK-cell-mediated cytotoxicity activated by naturally acquired infection in the mouse. *Int. J. Cancer, 24,* 688-699.

Clarke, M.D. (1983) The effect of stress on tumor induction. Toxicology Forum Annual Winter Meeting, February 21-23. Washington, D.C.

Clayson, D.B. (1962). Testing chemicals for carcinogenic activity I. Methods. In *Chemical Carcinogenesis* pp. 55-85, J. and A. Churchill, London.

Clayson, D.B. (1975). The chemical induction of cancer. In *Biology of Cancer* (E.J. Ambrose and F.J.C. Roe, eds.), pp. 163-179, Ellis Horwood Limited, England.

Clayson, D.B. (1979). Bladder carcinogenesis in rats and mice: possibility of artifacts. *National Cancer Institute Monograph Series, 52,* 519-524.

Clayson, D.B. (1981). Carcinogens and carcinogenesis enhancers. *Mutat. Res., 86,* 217-229.

Clayson, D.B. (1983). Trans-species and trans-tissue extrapolation in carcinogenicity assays. In *Organ and Species Specificity in Chemical Carcinogenesis* (R. Lengenbach, S. Nesnow and J.M. Rice, eds.), Plenum Press, New York.

Clayson, D.B. and Garner, R.C. (1976). Carcinogenic aromatic amines and related compounds. In *Chemical Carcinogens* (C.E. Searle, ed.), pp. 366-461, American Chemical Society, Washington.

Clayson, D.B., Krewski, D. and Munro, I.C. (1983). The power and interpretation of the carcinogenicity bioassay. *Reg. Toxicol. Pharmacol., 3,* 329-348.

Clifton, K.H. and Sridharin, B.N. (1975). Endocrine factor and tumor growth. In *Cancer: A Comprehensive Treatise* (F.F. Becker, ed.), Vol.3, pp. 249-286, Plenum Press, New York.

Clive, D., Johnson, K., Spector, J., Barson, A. and Brown, M. (1979). Validation and characterization of the L5178/TK+/-mouse lymphoma mutagen assay system. *Mutat. Res., 59*, 61-108.

Clive, D., and Specter, T.F.S. (1975). Laboratory procedure for assessing specific locus mutations at the TK locus in cultured L5178 mouse lymphoma cells. *Mutat. Res., 31*, 17-29.

Cohen, G.M., Bracken, W.M., Iyer, P.R., Berry, D.L., Selkirk, J.K. and Slaga, T.J. (1979a). Anticarcinogenic effects of 2,3,7,8-tetrachlorodibenzo-p-dioxin on benzo(a)-pyrene and 7,12-dimethylbenz(a)anthracene tumor initiation and its relationship to DNA binding. *Cancer Res., 39*, 4027-4033.

Cohen, S.M., Arai, M., Jacobs, J.B., Friedell, G.H. (1979b). Promoting effect of saccharin and DL-tryptophan in urinary bladder carcinogenesis. *Cancer Res., 39*, 1207-1217.

Cohen, A.J. and Grasso, P. (1981). Review of the hepatic response to hypolipidemic drugs in rodents and assessment of its toxicological significance to man. *Food Cosmet. Toxicol., 19*, 585-605.

Coleman, W.E., and Tardiff, R.G. (1979). Contaminant levels in animal feeds used for toxicity studies. *Arch. Environ. Contam. Toxicol., 8*, 693-702.

Connolly, J.G., Rider, W.D., Rosenbaum, J. and Chapman, A. (1978). Relation between the use of artificial sweeteners and bladder cancer. *Can. Med. Assoc. J., 119*, 408.

Coombs, M.M. and Croft, C.J. (1966). Carcinogenic derivatives of cyclopenta(a)phen-anthrene. *Nature (London), 210*, 1281-1282.

Cooper, G.M. (1982). Cellular transforming genes. *Science, 218*, 801-806.

Cooper, J.A., Saracci, R. and Cole, P. (1979). Describing the validity of carcinogen screening tests. *Br. J. Cancer, 39*, 87-89.

Cotruvo, J.A., Simmon, V.F. and Spanggord, R.J. (1977). Investigation of mutagenic effects of products of ozonation reactions in water. *Ann. N.Y. Acad. Sci., 298*, 124-140.

Coulston, F., McChesney, E.W. and Golberg, L. (1975). Long- term administration of artificial sweeteners to the rhesus monkey. *Food Cosmet. Toxicol., 13*, 297-300.

Cox, W.I., Holbrook, N.J. and Friedman, H. (1983). Mechanism of glucocorticoid action on murine natural killer cell activity. *J. Natl. Cancer Inst., 71*, 973-981.

Craddock, V.M. and Frei, J.V. (1974). Induction of liver cell adenomata in the rat by a single treatment with N-methyl-N-nitrosourea given at various times after partial hepatectomy. *Br. J. Cancer, 30*, 503-511.

Daniel, J.W. (1963). The metabolism of [36]Cl-labelled trichloroethylene and tetra-chloroethylene in the rat. *Biochem. Pharmacol, 12*, 795-802.

Davison, C., Scrime, M. and Edelson, J. (1977). Species differences in the metabolism of hycanthone. *Arch. Int. Pharmacodyn. Ther., 230*, 4.

Dean, B.J. (1978). Genetic toxicology of benzene, toluene, xylenes and phenols. *Mutat. Res., 47*, 75-97.

Dean, J.H., Luster, M.I., Boorman, G.A. and Lauer, L.D. (1982). Procedures available to examine the immunotoxicity of chemicals and drugs. *Pharmacol. Rev., 34*(1), 137-147.

De Clerca, E., Zhans, Zhen-Xi, Hussen, K. and Leyten, R. (1982). Inhibitory effect of interferon on the growth of spontaneous mammary tumors in mice. *J. Natl. Cancer Inst., 69*, 653-657.

Dees, J.H., Masters, B.S., Muller-Eberhard, U. and Johnson, E.F.(1982). Effect of 2,3,7,8-tetrachlorodibenzo-p-dioxin and phenobarbital on the occurrence and distribution of four cytochrome P-450 isozymes in rabbit kidney, lung and liver. *Cancer Res.*, 42, 1423-1432.

Deichmann, W.B. and McDonald, W.E. (1977). Organochlorine pesticides and liver cancer deaths in the United States. 1930-1972. *Ecotoxicol. Environ. Saf.*, 1, 89-110.

Dejana, E., Cerlette, C., De Castellarnau, C., Livio, N., Galletti, F., Latini, R. and De Gaetano, G. (1982). Salicylate-aspirin interaction in the rat. *J. Clin. Invest.*, 68, 1108-1112.

de la Iglesia, F. and Farber, E. (1981). Hepatocarcinogenesis of hypolipidemic agents. In *Organ Directed Toxicities Chemical Indices and Mechanisms* (IUPAC) (S. Brown and D. Davies, eds.), pp. 175-182, Pergamon Press, Oxford, New York.

de la Iglesia, F. and Farber, E. (1983). Hypolipidemics carcinogenicity and extrapolation of experimental results for human safety assessments. *Toxicol. Pathol. 10*, 152-170.

del Cerro, M., Grover, D.A., Monjan, A.A., Pfau, C.J. and Dematte, J.E. (1982). Chronic retinitis in rats infected as neonates with lymphocytic choriomeningitis virus: a clinical, histopathologic and electroretinographic study. *Invest. Ophthalmol. Vis. Sci., 23*, 697-714.

Demers, D.M., Fukushima, S. and Cohen, S.M. (1981). Effect of sodium saccharin and L-tryptophan on rat urine during bladder carcinogenesis. *Cancer Res., 41*, 108-112.

Dempster, A.P., Selwyn, M.R. and Weeks, J. (1983). Combining historical and randomized controls for assessing trends in proportions. *J. Am. Stat. Assoc., 78*, 221-227.

de Serres, F.J. (1980). The international program for the evaluation of short-term tests for carcinogenicity. In *The Predictive Value of In Vitro Short-Term Screening Test in Carcinogenicity Evaluation* (G.M. Williams, R. Kroes, H.W. Waaijers and K.W. van de Poll, eds.), Elsevier/North Holland, Amsterdam.

de Serres, F.J., and Ashby, J., (1981a). Selection, preparation, and purity of the test chemicals. *Prog. Mutat. Res., 1*, 8-15.

de Serres, F.J., and Ashby, J. (1981b). Evaluation of short-term tests for carcinogens. In *Progress in Mutation Research*, Elsevier/North Holland, Amsterdam.

Diala, E., Mittwoch, U. and Wilkie, D. (1980). Antimitochondrial effects of thioacetamide and ethylenethiourea in human and yeast cell culture. *Br. J. Cancer, 42*, 112.

Dia Mayorca, Greenblatt, M., Trauthen, T., Soller, A. and Giordano, R. (1973). Malignant transformation of BHK_{21} clone cells *in vitro* by nitrosamines - a conditional state. *Proc. Natl. Sci. Acad. U.S.A., 70*, 46-49.

Diamond, L.O'Brien, T.G. and Baird, W.M. (1980). Tumor promoters and the mechanism of tumor promotion. *Adv. Cancer Res., 32*, 1-74.

Diamond, L., O'Brien, T.G. and Rovera, G. (1978). Tumor promoters: effects of proliferation and differentiation of cells in culture. *Life Sci., 23*, 1979-1988.

Diaz, M., Fijtman, N., Carricarte, V., Braier, L. and Diez, J. (1979). Effect of benzene and its metabolites on SCE in human lymphocytes cultures. *In Vitro, 15*(3), 172.

Diaz, M., Reiser, A., Braier, L. and Diez, J. (1980). Studies on benzene mutagenesis. I. The micronucleus test. *Experientia, 36,* 297-299.

DiGiovanni, J., Viaje, A., Berry, D.L., Slaga, T.J. and Juchau, M.R.(1977). Tumor-initiating ability of 2,3,7,8-tetrachlorodibenzo-p-dioxin (TCDD) and arochlor 1254 in the two-stage system of mouse skin carcinogenesis. *Bull. Environ. Contam. Toxicol., 18,* 552-557.

DiPaola, T.A., Donnovan, P. and Nelson, R. (1979). Quantitative studies of *in vitro* transformation by chemical carcinogens. *J. Natl. Cancer Inst., 4,* 867-876.

Doll, R. (1979). Epidemiological enquiry. Power and limitations. In *Environmental Carcinogenesis: Occurrences, Risk Evaluation and Mechanism* (P. Emmelot and E. Krieb, eds.), Elsevier/North Holland, Amsterdam.

Doll, R. and Peto, R. (1981). *The Causes of Cancer: Quantitative Estimates of Avoidable Risks of Cancer in the United States Today.* Oxford University Press, Oxford.

Dreyfus, J., Shaw, J.M. and Ross, J.J. (1978). Absorption of the $\propto$-adrenergic agent nadolol by mice, rats, hamsters, rabbits, dogs, monkeys and man: an unusual species difference. *Xenobiotica, 8,* 503.

Dunkel, V., (1979). Personal communication.

Dunkel, V., (1981). Personal communication.

Dunkel, V.C., and Simmon, V.F. (1980). Mutagenic activity of chemicals previously tested for carcinogenicity in the National Cancer Institute Bioassay Program. In *Molecular and Cellular Aspects of Carcinogen Screening Tests* (R. Montesano, J. Bartsch and L. Tomatis, eds.), *27,* pp. 283-302, International Agency for Research on Cancer, Lyon.

Durham, W.F., Ortega, P. and Hayes, W.J., Jr. (1963). The effect of various dietary levels of DDT on liver function, cell morphology and DDT storage in the rhesus monkey. *Arch. Int. Pharmacodyn. Ther., 141,* 111-129.

Edwards, G.S., Fox, J.G., Policastro, P., Goff, U., Wolff, M.N. and Fine, D.H. (1979). Volatile nitrosamine contamination of laboratory animal diets. *Cancer Res., 39,* 1837-1858.

Egan, H., Goulding, R., Roburn, J., Tatton, J. (1965). Organochlorine pesticide residues in human fat and human milk. *Br. Med. J., 2,* 66-69.

Ehrlich, R., Efrati, M., Malatzky, E., Shochat, L., Bar-eyan, A. and Witz, I.P. (1983). Natural host defense during oncogenesis. NK activity and dimethylbenzanthracene carcinogenesis. *Int. J. Cancer, 31,* 67-73.

Elek, S.J. and Jambor, E. (1978). The effects of hypolipidemic agents on the hepatic drug metabolism of the rat. In *Proceedings of the First International Congress on Toxicology: Toxicology as a Predictive Science* (G.L. Plaa and W.A.M. Duncan, eds.), p. 641, Academic Press, New York

Epstein, S. (1970) cited by S. S. Epstein in *Int. J. Environ. Studies, 2,* 291 and *3,* 13 (1972).

Epstein, S.S. and Shafner, H. (1968). Chemical mutagens in the human environment. *Nature, 219,* 385-387.

Epstein S.S., Arnold, E., Andrea, J., Bass, W. and Bishop, Y. (1972). Detection of chemical mutagens by the dominant lethal assay in the mouse. *Toxicol. Appl. Pharmacol.* 23, 288-325.

Eva, A. (1982). Cellular genes analogous to retroviral oncogenes are transcribed in human tumor cells. *Nature, 295,* 116-119.

Evans, C.H. (1983). Lymphokines, homeostasis, and carcinogenesis. *J. Natl. Cancer Inst., 71,* 153-257.

Evans, C.H., DiPaolo, J.A., Heinbaugh, J.A. and Demarinis, A.J. (1982). Immuno-modulation of the lymphoresponsive phases of carcinogenesis: mechanisms of natural immunity. *J. Natl. Cancer Inst., 69,* 737-740.

Fahring, R. (1974). Comparative mutagenicity studies with pesticides. In *Chemical Carcinogensis Essays*, p. 161, International Agency for Research on Cancer, Lyon.

Farber, E. and Solt, D. (1978). A new liver model for the study of promotion. In *Mechanisms of Tumor Promotion Cocarcinogenesis* (T.J. Slaga, R.K. Boutwell and A. Sivak, eds.), Vol. 2., pp. 443-448, Raven Press, New York.

Federal Register (1980).Occupational Safety and Health Administration (OSHA) Department of Labor. *Identification, Classification and Regulation of Potential Occupational Carcinogens.*, 45, 50002-5296; Proposed Amendments to the OSHA Cancer Policy., *46,* 7402.

Federal Register (1978a). Non-clinical laboratory studies. Good laboratory regulations, *43,* 59986-60024.

Federal Register (1978b). Oncogenicity studies, *43*(163), 37379-37382.

Filov, V.A., Golubev, A.A., Linblina, E.I. and Tolokontsev, N.A. (eds.) (1979). The toxic effect as a result of interaction between the poison and the living organism. In *Quantitative Toxicology*, John Wiley and Sons, New York.

Fish, D.C., Demarais, J.T., Djurickovic, D.B. and Huebner, R.J. (1981). Prevention of 3-methylcholanthrene-induced fibrosarcomas in rats pre-inoculated with endogenous rat retrovirus. *Proc. Natl. Acad. Sci. U.S.A., 78,* 2526-2527.

Fishbein, L. (1979). Overview of some aspect of occurrence, formation, and analysis of nitrosamines. *Sci. Total Environ., 13,* 157-188.

Fisher, P.B., Miranada, A.F., Mufson, R.A., Weinstein, L.S., Fujiki, H., Sugimura, T. and Weinstein, I.B. (1982). Effects of teleocidin and the phorbol ester tumor promoters on cell transformation, differentiation, and phospholipid metabolism. *Cancer Res., 42,* 2829-2835.

Fitzhugh, O.G., Nelson, A.A. and Frawley, J.P. (1951). A comparison of the chronic toxicities of synthetic sweetening agents. *J. Am. Pharmacol. Assoc., 40,* 583-586.

Flamm, G. (1983). FDA viewpoint on problem tumors. *Proceedings, The Toxicology Forum 1983 Annual Winter Meeting*, pp. 367-375, February 21-23, Washington, D.C.

Foley, P.D., Becking, G., Muller, J., Goyer, R.A., Falk, H.L. and Chernoff, N. (1977). Report to the Great Lakes Research Advisory Board of the International Joint Commission on the Health Implications of NTA.

FSC (Food Safety Council) (1978). Scientific Committee. Proposed system for food safety assessment. *Food Cosmet. Toxicol., 16* (Suppl. 2), 1-136.

Fox, J.G. (1977). Clinical assessment of laboratory rodents on long-term bioassay studies. *J. Environ. Pathol. Toxicol., 1*, 199-226.

Fox, J.G., Thibert, P., Arnold, D.L., Krewski, D.R. and Grice H.C. (1979). Toxicology studies II. The laboratory animal. *Food Cosmet. Toxicol., 17*, 661-675.

Frank, L. and Massaro, D. (1980). Oxygen toxicity. *Am. J. Med., 69*, 117.

Franklin, R.A., and Aldridge, A. (1976). Pharmacokinetics and metabolism of the new analgesic meptazinol in rats and patas monkey. *Xenobiotica, 6*, 499.

Frith, C.H. and Jaques, W.E. (1974). Histopathologic changes in mice fed 2-acetyl-aminofluorene in a chronic study. (Abstract) *Toxicol. Appl. Pharmacol., 29*, 106.

Fukuda, K., Matsushita, H., Sakabe, H. and Takemoto, K. (1981). Carcinogenicity of benzyl chloride, benzal chloride, benzotrichloride and benzoyl chloride in mice by skin application. *Gann, 72*, 655-664.

Fukushima, S. and Cohen, S.M. (1980). Saccharin induced hyperplasia of the rat urinary bladder. *Cancer Res., 40*, 734-736.

Fukushima, S., Friedell, G.H., Jacobs, J.B. and Cohen, S.M. (1981). Effect of L-tryptophan and sodium saccharin on urinary tract carcinogenesis initiated by N-[4-(5-nitro-2-furyl)-2-thiazolyl] formamide. *Cancer Res., 41*, 3100-3103.

Galli, M.C., DeGiovanni, C., Nicoletti, G., Grilli, S., Nanni, P., Prodi, G., Gola, G., Riocchetta, R. and Orlandi, C. (1981). The occurrence of multiple steroid hormone receptors in disease-free and neoplastic human ovary. *Cancer, 47, 1297-1302.*

Garattini, S., Bartosek, I., Donelli, N.G. and Spreafico, F. (1975). Interaction of anticancer agents with other drugs. In *Pharmacological Basis of Cancer Chemotherapy*. pp. 565-593, Symposium on Fundamental Cancer Research, 27, M.D. Anderson Hospital and Tumor Institute, Houston, Texas.

Garlinghouse, L.E. and Van Hoosier, G.L. (1978). Studies on adjuvant-induced arthritis, tumor transplantability and serologic response to bovine serum albumin in Sendai virus-infected rats. *Am. J. Vet. Res., 39*, 297-300.

Gart, J.J., Chu, K.C. and Tarone, R.E. (1979). Statistical issues in interpretation of chronic bioassay tests for carcinogenicity. *J. Natl. Cancer Inst., 62*, 957-974.

Gehring, P.J. and Blau, G.E. (1977). Mechanisms of carcinogenesis: dose response. *J. Environ. Pathol. Toxicol., 1*, 163-179.

Gehring, P.J., Watanabe, P.G. and Blau, G.E. (1979). Risk assessment of environmental carcinogens utilizing pharmacokinetic parameters. *Ann. N.Y. Acad. Sci., 329*, 137.

Geiger, L.E., and Neal, R.A. (1981). Mutagenicity testing of 2,3,7,8-tetrachlorodibenzo-p-dioxin in histidine auxotrophs of *Salmonella typhimurium. Toxicol. Appl. Pharmacol., 59*, 125-129.

Gelboin, H.F., (1976). Mechanics of induction of drug metabolism enzymes. In *Fundamentals of Drug Metabolism and Drug Disposition* (B.N. LaDu, H.G. Mandel and E.L. Way, eds.), p. 279, Williams and Wilkins, Baltimore.

Gerner-Smidt, P. and Friedrich, U. (1978). The mutagenic effect of benzene, toluene and xylene studied by the SCE technique. *Mutat. Res., 58*, 313-316.

Gandilhon, P., Melancon, R.M., Gandilhon, F., Djiane, J. and Kelly, P.A. (1983). Prolactin receptors in N-nitroso-N-methylurea-induced rat mammary tumors: relationship to tumor age and down-regulation in short-term explant cultures. *J. Natl. Cancer Inst., 70*, 105-109.

Gilbert, P., Saint-Ruf, G., Poncelet, F. and Mercier, M. (1980). Genetic effects of chlorinated anilines and azobenzenes on *Salmonella typhimurium*. *Arch. Environ. Contam. Toxicol., 9*, 533-541.

Gillette, J.R. (1977). The phenomenon of species variations: problems and opportunities. In *Drug Metabolism from Microbes to Man* (D.V. Parke and R.L. Smith, eds.), pp. 147-168, Taylor and Francis, London.

Gillette, J.R. (1976). Application of pharmacokinetic principles in the extrapolation of animal data to humans. *Clin. Toxicol., 9*, 709.

Gillette, J.R. and Mitchell, J.R. (1975). In *Handbuch der Experimentellen Pharmakologie* (O. Eichler, A. Farah, H. Herken and A.D. Welch, eds.), pp. 359-381, Springer-Verlag, Berlin.

Glazko, A.J., Dil, W.A. and Wolf, L.M. (1952). Metabolic disposition of chloramphenicol in the rat. *J. Pharmacol. Exper. Ther., 104*, 452.

Gold, B., Leuschen, T., Brunk, G. and Gingell, R. (1981). Metabolism of a DDT metabolite via a chloroepoxide. *Chem.-Biol. Interact., 35*, 159-176.

Goldfarb, S. (1976). Sex hormones and hepatic neoplasia. *Cancer Res., 36*, 2584-2588.

Goldstein, R.S., Hook, J.B. and Bond, J.T. (1978). Renal tubular transport of saccharin. *J. Pharmacol. Exp. Ther., 204*, 690-695.

Goodman, D.G.,Ward, J.M., Squire, R.A., Paxton, M.B., Reichardt, W.D., Chu, K.C. and Linhart, M.S. (1980). Neoplastic and nonneoplastic lesions in aging and Osborne-Mendel rats. *Toxicol. Appl. Pharmacol., 55*, 433-447.

Gorelik, E. and Herberman, R.B. (1981a). Inhibition of the activity of mouse natural killer cells by urethane. *J. Natl. Cancer Inst., 66*, 543-548.

Gorelik, E. and Herberman, R.B. (1981b). Susceptibility of various strains of mice to urethane-induced tumors and depressed natural killer cell activity. *J. Natl. Cancer Inst., 67*, 1317-1322.

Gorelik, E., Wiltrout, R.H., Okumura, K., Habu, S. and Herberman, R.B. (1982). Role of NK cells in the control of metastatic spread and growth of tumor cells in mice. *Int. J. Cancer, 30*, 107-112.

Gori, G. (1978). Role of diet and nutrition in cancer cause, prevention and treatment. *Bull. Cancer, 15*, 115-126.

Goyer, R.A.,Falk, H.L., Hogan, M., Feldman, D.D. and Richter,W. (1981). Renal tumors in rats given trisodium nitrilotriacetic acid in drinking water for two years. *J. Natl. Cancer Inst., 66*, 869.

Grafstrom, R., Stohs, S.J., Burke, M.D., Moldeus, P. and Orrenius, S. (1977). Benzo(a)-pyrene metabolism by microsomes and isolated epithelial cells from rat small intestine. In

Microsomes and Drug Oxidations (V. Ullrich, A. Hildebrandt, I. Roots, R.W. Estabrook and A.H. Conney, eds.), p. 667, Pergamon Press, New York.

Graham, S., Davis, K., Hansen, W. and Graham, C. (1975). Effects of prolonged ethylenethiourea ingestion on the thyroid of the rat. *Food Cosmet. Toxicol., 13*, 493-449.

Graham, S., Hansen, W., Davis, K. and Perry, H. (1973). Effects of one-year administration of ethylenethiourea upon thyroid function of the rat. *Bull. Environ. Contam. Toxicol. (U.S.), 7*, 19.

Grasso, P. and Hardy, J. (1975). Strain difference in natural incidence and response to carcinogens. In *Mouse Hepatic Neoplasia* (W.H. Butler and P.M. Newberne, eds.), pp. 111-132, Elsevier/North Holland, Amsterdam.

Green, S., and Moreland, F.S. (1975). Cytogenetic evaluation of several dioxins in the rat. *Toxicol. Appl. Pharmacol., 33*, 161 (abstract).

Green, U., Schneider T., Deutsch-Wenzel, R., Brune, H. and Althoff, J. (1980). Syncarcinogenic action of saccharin or sodium cyclamate in the induction of bladder tumors in MNU- pretreated rats. *Food Cosmet. Toxicol., 18*, 575-579.

Greenblatt, W. and Lijinsky, W. (1974). Carcinogenesis and chronic toxicity of nitrilotriacetic acid in Swiss mice. *J. Natl. Cancer Inst., 52*, 1123.

Greenman, D.L., Bryant, P., Kodell, R.L. and Sheldon, W. (1982). Influence of cage shelf level on retinal atrophy in mice. *Lab. Anim. Sci., 32*, 353-356.

Greim, H., Bimbors, D., Egert, G.,Gögfelmann,W. and Krämer, M. (1977a). Mutagenicity and chromosomal aberrations as an analytical tool for *in vitro* detection of mammalian enzyme-mediated formation of reactivated metabolites. *Arch. Toxicol., 39*, 159-169.

Greim, H., Bonse, G. and Henschler, D. (1977b). Mutagenicity of vinyl chloride and other chlorinated ethylenes. *Leberschaeden Vinylchloride: Vinylchlorid-Kr.,[Wiss. Tag.], 2*, 36-40.

Grice, H.C. (1978). The acceptance of risk benefit decisions. In *Chemical Toxicology of Foods* (C.L. Galli, R. Pavletti and G. Vettorazzi, eds.), pp. 33-45, Elsevier/North Holland, Amsterdam.

Grice, H.C. and Burek, J. (1983). Age-associated (geriatric) pathology: its impact on long-term toxicity studies. In *Current Issues in Toxicology* (H.C. Grice, ed.), pp. 57-95, Springer-Verlag, New York.

Grice, H.C., Munro, I.C., Krewski, D.R. and Blumenthal, H. (1980). *In utero* exposure in chronic toxicity/carcinogenicity studies. *Food Cosmet. Toxicol., 19*, 373-379.

Griesemer, R.A. and Cueto, C., Jr., (1980). Toward a classification scheme for degrees of experimental evidence for the carcinogenicity of chemicals for animals. In *Molecular and Cellular Aspects of Carcinogen Screening Tests*. (R. Montesano, H. Bartsch and L. Tomatis, eds.), pp. 259-281, International Agency for Research on Cancer, Lyon.

Griffin D.E. and Hill, W.E. (1978). *In vitro* breakage of plasmid DNA by mutagens and pesticides. *Mutat. Res., 52*, 161-169.

Grignolo, A., Orzalesi, N., Castellazzo, R. and Vittone, P. (1969). Retinal damage by visible light in albino rats. *Ophthalmologica, 157*, 43-59.

Grosch, D.S. and Valcovic, L.R. (1967). Chlorinated hydrocarbon insecticides are not mutagenic in bracon hebetor tests. *J. Econ. Entomol., 60*, 1177-1179.

Grunberger, D. and Weinstein, I.B. (1979). Conformational changes in nucleic acids modified by chemical carcinogens. In *Chemical Carcinogens and DNA* (P.L. Grover, ed.), pp. 59-93, CRC Press, Boca Raton.

Günther, T.M., Fyst, J.M. and Nebert, D.W. (1979). 2,3,7,8-tetrachlorodibenzo-p-dioxin: covalent binding of reactive metabolic intermediates principally to protein *in vitro. Pharmacology, 19*, 12-22.

Hamilton, T. (1969). Influence of environmental light and melatonin upon mammary tumor induction. *Br. J. Surg., 56*, 764-766.

Hamilton, T.C., Davies, P. and Griffiths, K. (1982). Estrogen receptor-like binding in the surface germinal epithelium of the rat ovary. *J. Endocrinol., 95*, 377-385.

Hamilton, T.C., Davies, P. and Griffiths, K. (1983a). Steroid-hormone receptor status of the normal and neoplastic ovarian surface germinal epithelium. In *Factors Regulating Ovarian Function* (G.S. Greenwald and P.F. Terranova, eds.), pp.81-85, Raven Press, New York.

Hamilton, T.C., Young R.C., McKoy, W., Grotzinger, K.R., Green, J.A., Chu, E.W., Whang-Peng, J., Rogan, A.M., Green, W.R. and Ozols, R.F. (1983b). Characterization of a human ovarian carcinoma cell line (NIH:OVCAR-3)[1] with androgen and estrogen receptors. *Cancer Res., 43*, 5379-5389.

Hanefeld, M., Kemmer, C., Leonhardt, W. and Jaross, W. (1977).Der effekt der regardin (CPIB)-therapie von hyperlipoproteinamien (HLP) auf die leber. *Dtsch. Gesundheitswes., 32*, 2267.

Hanefeld, M., Kemmer, C., Leonhardt, W., Kunze, K.D., Jaross, W.and Haller, H. (1980). Effects of p-chlorophenoxyisobutyric acid (CPIB) on the human liver. *Atherosclerosis, 36*, 159-172.

Hanna, M.G. and Fidler, I.J. (1980). Role of natural killer cells in the destruction of circulating tumor emboli. *J. Natl. Cancer Inst., 65*, 801-809.

Hanna, M.G., Netteshiem, P., Richter, C.B. and Tennant, R.W. (1973). The variable influence of host microflora and intercurrent infections on immunological competence and carcinogenesis. *Isr. J. Med. Sci., 9*, 229-238.

Harris, M.W., Moore, J.A., Vos, J.G. and Gupta, B.N. (1973). General biological effects of TCDD (2,3,7,8,-tetrochlorodibenzo-p-dioxin) in laboratory animals. *Environ. Health Perspect., 5*, 101-109.

Hart, L.G. and Fauts, J.R. (1963). Effects of acute and chronic DDT administration on hepatic microsomal drug metabolism in the rat. *Proc. Soc. Exp. Biol. Med. U.S.A., 114*, 388-392.

Haseman, J.K. (1983). Patterns of tumor incidence in two-year cancer bioassay feeding studies in Fischer 344 rats. *Fund. Appl. Toxicol., 3*, 1-9.

Haseman, J.K. and Kupper, L. (1979). Analysis of dichotomous response data from certain toxicological experiments. *Biometrics, 35*, 281.

Hatch, T.F. and Gross, P. (1964). *Pulmonary Deposition of Inhaled Aerosols*. Academic Press, New York.

Hattula, M.L., Ikkala, J. Isomki, M., Määttä, K. and Arstila, A.U. (1976). Chlorinated hydrocarbon residues (PCB and DDT) in human liver, adipose tissue and brain in Finland. *Acta Pharmacol. Toxicol., 39*, 545-554.

Health and Welfare Canada (1975). *Testing of Chemicals for Carcinogenicity, Mutagenicity and Teratogenicity*. pp. 2-31, Health and Welfare Canada, Ottawa.

Health Council of the Netherlands (1978). *Report on the Evaluation of the Carcinogenicity of Chemical Substances*, pp. 3-4, Government Publishing Office, The Hague.

Health Council of the Netherlands (1980). *The Evaluation of the Carcinogenicity of Chemical Substances*. Report submitted by a committee of the Health Council of the Netherlands. Ministry of Health and Environmental Protection, Leidschendam, The Netherlands.

Hecker, E., Fusenig, N.E., Kunz, W., Marks, F. and Thielmann, H.W. (eds.) (1982). Cocarcinogenesis and biological effects of tumor promoters. In *Carcinogenesis* Vol. 7., Raven Press, New York.

Herberman, R.B. and Holden, H.T. (1978). Natural cell-mediated immunity. *Adv. Cancer Res., 27*, 305-377.

Herberman, R.B. and Ortaldo, J.R. (1981). Natural killer cells: their roles in defenses against disease. *Science, 214*, 24-30.

Hess, R., Staübli, W. and Reiss, W. (1965). Nature of the hepatomegalic effect produced by ethylchlorophenoxyisobutyrate in the rat. *Nature (London), 208*, 856-858.

Heywood, R. (1982). Histopathological and laboratory assessment of visual dysfunction. *Environ. Health Perspect., 44*, 35-45.

Heywood, R., Sortwell, R.J., Noel, P.R.B., Street, D.E., Prentice, D.E., Roe, F.J.C., Wadsworth, P.R. and van Abbé, N.J. (1979). Safety evaluation of toothpaste containing chloroform. III. Long term study in beagle dogs. *J. Environ. Pathol. Toxicol., 2*, 835-851.

Hicks, R.M. and Chowaniec, J. (1977). The importance of synergy between weak carcinogens in the induction of bladder cancer in experimental animals and humans. *Cancer Res., 37*, 2943-2949.

Hicks, R.M., Chowaniec, J. and Wakefield, J.St.J. (1978). Experimental induction of bladder tumors by a two-stage system. In *Mechanism of Tumor Promotion and Cocarcinogenesis* (T.J. Slaga, R.K. Boutwell and A. Sivak, eds.), Vol. 2, pp. 475-490, Raven Press, New York.

Hicks, R.M., Wakefield, J.St.J. and Chowaniec, J. (1975). Evaluation of a new model to detect bladder carcinogens or cocarcinogens: results obtained with saccharin, cyclamate and cyclophosphamide. *Chem.-Biol. Interact.* 11, 225-233.

Hill, M.J. (1980). Bacterial metabolism and human carcinogenesis. *Br. Med. Bull., 36*, 89-94.

Hisano, G. and Hanna, N. (1982). Murine lymph node natural killer cells: regulatory mechanisms of activation or suppression. *J. Natl. Cancer Inst.*, 69, 665-671.

Hite, M., Pecharo, M., Smith, I. and Thornton, S. (1980). Effect of benzene in the micronucleus test. *Mutat. Res., 77*, 149-155.

Hodgson, E. (1980). *Introduction to Biochemical Toxicology* (E. Hodgson and F.E. Gutherie, eds.), pp. 143-161, Elsevier/North Holland, New York.

Hoel, D.G. (1983). Conditional two-sample tests with historical control. In *Contributions to Statistics. Essays in Honor of Norman L. Johnson* (P.K. Sen, ed.), pp. 229-236, Elsevier/North Holland, Amsterdam.

Hollstein, M., McCann, J., Angelosanto, F.A., and Nichols, W. (1979). Short-term tests for carcinogens and mutagens. *Mutat. Res., 65*, 133-226.

Hoover, R. (1980). Saccharin--bitter aftertaste? *New Engl. J. Med., 302*, 573.

Hoover, R.N. and Strasser, P.H. (1980). Artificial sweeteners and human bladder cancer, preliminary results. *Lancet, 1*, 837-840.

Howard, R.J., Notkins, A.L. and Mergenhagen, S.E. (1969). Inhibition of cellular immune reactions in mice infected with lactic dehydrogenase virus. *Nature, 221*, 873-874.

Howe, G.R., Burch, J.D., Miller, A.B., Cook, G.M., Esteve, J., Morrison B., Gordon, P., Chambers, L.W., Fodor, G. and Winsor, G.M. (1980). Tobacco use, occupation, coffee, various nutrients and bladder cancer. *J. Natl. Cancer Inst., 64*, 701-713.

Hughes, D.L., Bruce, R.D., Hart, R.W., Fishbein, L., Gaylor, D.W., Smith, J.M. and Carlton, W.W. (1983). A report on the workshop on biological and statistical implications of the ED_{01} study and related data bases. *Fund. Appl. Toxicol., 3*, 129-136.

Hussain, S., Ehrenberg, L., Lofroth, G. and Gejvall, T. (1972). Mutagenic effects of TCDD (2,3,7,8,-tetrochlorodibenzo-p-dioxin) on bacterial systems. *Ambio., 1*, 32-33.

Ikeda, M. (1977). Metabolism of trichloroethylene and tetrachloroethylene in human subjects. *Environ. Health Perspect., 21*, 239-245.

Ikeda, M. and Imamura, T. (1973). Biological half-life of trichloroethylene and tetra-chloroethylene in human subjects. *Int. Arch. Arbeitsmed., 31*, 209-244.

Ikeda, M., Koizumi, A., Watanabe, T., Endo, A. and Sato, K. (1980). Cytogenetic and cytokinetic investigations on lymphocytes from workers occupationally exposed to tetrachloroethylene. *Toxicol. Lett., 5*, 251-256.

Illett, K.F., Reid, W.D., Sipes, I.G. and Krishna, G. (1973). Chloroform toxicity in mice: correlation of renal and hepatic necrosis with covalent binding of metabolites to tissue macromolecules. *Exp. Mol. Pathol., 19*, 215-229.

Illing, H.P.A. and Fromson, J.M. (1978). Species differences in the disposition and metabolism of 6,11-dihydro-11-oxodibenz(be)oxepin-2-acetic acid (isoxepac) in rat, rabbit, dog, rhesus monkey and man. *Drug. Metab. Dispos., 6*, 510-517.

IARC (International Agency for Research on Cancer) (1972-1980). *Monographs on the Evaluation of Carcinogenic Risk of Chemicals to Man.* Volumes 1-20, IARC, Lyon.

IARC (International Agency for Research on Cancer) (1972). *Oncogenesis and Herpes viruses.* IARC Scientific Publications, Lyon.

IARC (International Agency for Research on Cancer) (1974a). *Monographs on the Evaluation of Carcinogenic Risk of Chemicals to Man. Sex Hormones.* IARC, Lyon.

IARC (International Agency for Research on Cancer) (1974b). *Monographs on the Evaluation of Carcinogenic Risk of Chemicals to Man. Some Anti-thyroid and Related Substances, Nitroflurans and Industrial Chemicals.* IARC, Lyon.

IARC (International Agency for Research on Cancer) (1976a). *Screening Tests in Chemical Carcinogenesis*. IARC Scientific Publications, Lyon.

IARC (International Agency for Research on Cancer) (1976b). *Monographs on the Evaluation of Carcinogenic Risk of Chemicals to Man. Some Carbamates, Thiocarbamates and Carbazides*. IARC, Lyon.

IARC (International Agency for Research on Cancer) (1977). *Directory of On-Going Research in Cancer Epidemiology*. IARC Scientific Publications, Lyon.

IARC (International Agency for Research on Cancer) (1979a). *Monographs on the Evaluation of Carcinogenic Risk of Chemicals to Man. Supplement 1: Chemicals and Industrial Processes Associated with Cancer in Humans*. IARC, Lyon.

IARC (International Agency for Research on Cancer) (1979b). *Monographs on the Evaluation of Carcinogenic Risk of Chemicals to Man. Sex Hormones II*, pp. 401-427, IARC, Lyon.

IARC (International Agency for Research on Cancer) (1979c). *Monographs on the Evaluation of Carcinogenic Risk of Chemicals to Man. Some Halogenated Hydrocarbons: Tetrachloroethylene*. pp. 491-514, IARC, Lyon.

IARC (International Agency for Research on Cancer) (1980a). An evaluation of chemicals and industrial processes associated with cancer in humans based on human and animal data. *Cancer Res., 40*, 1-12.

IARC (International Agency for Research on Cancer) (1980b). *Monographs on the Evaluation of Carcinogenic Risk of Chemicals to Man. Supplement 2: Long-term and Short-term Screening Assays for Carcinogens: A Critical Appraisal*. IARC, Lyon.

IARC (International Agency for Research on Cancer) (1982) *Monographs on the Evaluation of Carcinogenic Risk of Chemicals to Man. Some Industrial Chemicals and Dyestuffs*. pp. 93-148, IARC, Lyon.

IARC (International Agency for Research on Cancer) (1983) *Approaches to Classifying Chemical Carcinogens According to Mechanisms of Action*. Technical Report 83/001, IARC Scientific Publications, Lyon.

ICPEMC (International Commission for the Protection of the Environment against Mutagens and Carcinogens) (1982). Committee 2, Final Report, Mutagenesis testing as an approach to carcinogenesis. *Mutat. Res., 99*, 93-91.

ICPEMC (International Commission for the Protection of the Environment against Mutagens and Carcinogens) (1983). Committee 1, Final Report, Recommendations for development of a genetic screening program. *Mutat. Res., 114*, 117-177.

IRLG (Interagency Regulatory Liaison Group) (1979). The scientific basis for identification of potential carcinogens and estimation of risks. Report of the Interagency Regulatory Liaison Group. *J. Natl. Cancer Inst., 63*, 241-268.

IRLG (Interagency Regulatory Liaison Group) (1980). Scientific basis for identification of potential carcinogens and estimation of risks. *Am. Rev. Public Health., 1*, 345-393.

Ioannides, C. and Parke, D.V. (1980). The metabolic activation and detoxification of mutagens and carcinogens. *Chem. Ind. 24*, 854.

Irons, R.D., Dent, J.G., Baker, T.S. and Rickert, D.E. (1980) Benzene is metabolized and covalently bound in bone marrow *in situ. Chem.-Biol. Interact., 30*, 241-245.

Ishidate, M., Jr., and Odashima, S. (1977). Chromosome tests with 134 compounds on Chinese hamster cells *in vitro* - a screening for chemical carcinogens. *Mutat. Res., 48*, 337-354.

Iverson, F., Khera, K. and Hierlihy, S. (1980). *In vivo* and *in vitro* metabolism of ethylenethiourea in the rat and cat. *Toxicol. Appl. Pharmacol., 52*, 16-21.

Jeffrey, A.M., Kinsohita, T., Santella, R.M., Grunberger, D., Katz, L. and Weinstein, I.B. (1980). The chemistry of polycyclic aromatic hydrocarbon-DNA adducts. In *Carcinogens: Fundamental Mechanisms and Environmental Effects* (B. Pullman, P.O.P. Ts'o and H. Gelboin, eds.), pp. 565-579, Reidel, Amsterdam.

Jones, C.A., Marlino, P.J., Lijinsky, W. and Huberman, E.(1981). The relationship between the carcinogenicity and mutagenicity of nitrosamines in a hepatocyte-mediated mutagenicity assay. *Carcinogenesis, 2*, 1075-1077.

Jones, W.I., Roback, L.A. and Taylor, J.M. (1971). The loss of food flavors from laboratory animals diets II. Effect of laboratory environment. *J. Assoc. Off. Anal. Chem., 54*, 42-26.

Jongen, W.M.F., Alink, G.M. and Koeman, J.H. (1978). Mutagenic effect of dichloromethane on *Salmonella typhimurium. Mutat. Res., 56*, 245-248.

Jongen, W.M.F., Lohman, P.H.M., Kottenhagen, M.J., Alink, G.M., Berends, F. and Lowman, J.H. (1981). Mutagenicity testing of dichloromethane in short-term mammalian test systems. *Mutat. Res., 81*, 203-213.

Jorgenson, T.A., Newell, G.A., Scharpf, L.G., Gribling, P., O'Brien, M. and Chu, D. (1975). Abstract # 5, Sixth Annual Meeting of the American Environmental Mutagen Society, p. 337.

Jori, A. and Caccia, S. (1975). Further studies on brain concentrations of amphetamine and its metabolites in strains of mice showing different sensitivity to pharmacological effects of amphetamine. *Pharm. Pharmacol., 27*, 886-888.

Jusko, W.J. and Levy, G. (1970). Pharmacokinetic evidence for saturable renal tubular reabsorption of riboflavin. *J. Pharmacol. Sci., 59*, 765.

Kahl, R., Friederici, D.E., Kahl, G.F., Ritter, W. and Krebs, R. (1980). Clotrimazole as an inhibitor of benzo[a]pyrene metabolite-DNA adduct formation *in vitro* and of microsomal mono-oxygenase activity. *Drug Metab. Dispos., 8*, 191-196.

Kakunaga, T. (1973). A quantitative system for assay of malignant transformation by chemical carcinogens using a clone derived from BALB/c 3T3. *Int. J. Cancer, 12*, 463-473.

Kalland, T. and Forsberg, J. (1983). 3-Methylcholanthrene: transient inhibition of the lytic step of mouse natural killer cells. *J. Natl. Cancer Inst., 71*, 385-390.

Kao, J., Bridges, J.W. and Faulkner, J.K. (1979) Metabolism of (14C) phenol by sheep, pig and rat. *Xenobiotica, 9*, 141.

Karre, K., Klein, G.O., Kiessling, R., Klein, G. and Roger, J.C. (1980). Low natural *in vivo* resistance to syngeneic leukemias in natural killer-deficient mice. *Nature, 284*, 624-626.

Kashyap, S.K., Nigam, S.K., Karnik, A.B., Gupta, R.C. and Chatterjee, S.K. (1977). Carcinogenicity of DDT (dichlorodiphenyltrichloroethane) in pure inbred Swiss mice. *Int. J. Cancer, 19*, 725-729.

Kawachi, T., Yahagi, T., Kada, T., Tazima, Y., Ishidate, M., Sasaki, M. and Sugiyama, T. (1980). Cooperative program on short-term assays for carcinogenicity. In *Molecular and Cellular Aspects of Carcinogen Screening Tests* (R. Montesano, H. Bartsch and L. Tomatis, eds.), pp.323-330, IARC Scientific Publications, Lyon.

Kawarjiri, K., Yonekawa, H., Hara, E. and Tagashira, Y. (1979). Activation of 2-acetylaminofluorene in the nuclei of rat liver. *Cancer Res., 39*, 1089-1093.

Kay, M.M.B., Mendoza, J., Hausman, S. and Dorsey, B. (1979). Age related changes in the immune system of mice of eight medium and long-lived strains and hybrids. II. Short and long-term effects of natural infection with parainfluenza type I virus (Sendai). *Mech. Aging Dev., 11*, 347-362.

Keck, G. (1981). Species difference in the pharmacokinetics of chemicals, correlations with toxicity. *Toxicol. Eur. Res., 3*, 207.

Keller, R. (1983). Host defense mechanisms against tumors as the principal targets of tumor promoters. *J. Cancer Res. Clin. Oncol., 105*, 203-211.

Kelloff, G.J., Peters, R.L., Donahoe, R.M., Ghazzouli, I., Sass, B., Nims, R.M. and Huebner, R.J. (1976). An approach to C-type virus immunoprevention of spontaneously occurring tumors in laboratory mice. *Cancer Res., 36*, 622-630.

Kennedy, G., Fancher, O.E., Calandra, J.C. and Keller, R.E. (1972). Metabolic fate of saccharin in the albino rat. *Food Cosmet. Toxicol., 10*, 143.

Kessler, I. (1970). Cancer mortality among diabetics. *J. Natl. Cancer Inst., 44*, 673-686.

Kessler, I. (1976). Non-nutritive sweeteners and human bladder cancer: preliminary findings. *J. Urol., 115*, 143-146.

Kessler, I. (1978). Saccharin, cyclamate, and human bladder cancer. *J. Am. Med. Assoc., 240*, 349-355.

Khera, K.S. and Ruddick, J.A. (1973). Polychlorodibenzo-p-dioxins: perinatal affects and the dominant lethal test in Wistar rats. Chlorodioxins-origin and fate. In *Advances in Chemistry*, Series N6-120 (E.H. Blair, ed.), pp. 70-84, American Chemical Society, Washington, D.C.

Kihlman, B.A. (1971). Root tips for studying the effects of chemicals in chromosomes in chemical mutagens. In *Chemical Mutagens: Principles and Methods for Their Detection*, (A. Hollander, ed.) Vol. 2, pp. 489-514, Plenum Press, New York.

Kinsilla, A.R. (1982). Elimination of metabolic cooperation and the induction of sister chromatid exchanges are not properties common to all promoting or co-carcinogenic agents. *Carcinogenesis, 3*, 499-503.

Kinsilla, A.R., and Radman, M. (1978). Tumor promoter induces sister chromatid exchanges: relevance to mechanisms of carcinogenesis. *Proc. Natl. Acad. Sci. U.S.A.*, 75, 6149.

Kirschbaum, A. and Strong, L.C. (1942). Influence of carcinogens on the age incidence of leukemia in the high leukemia F strain of mice. *Cancer Res., 2*, 841-845.

Klaassen, C.D. (1980). Absorption, distribution and excretion of toxicants. In *Toxicology: The Basic Science of Poisons* (J. Doull, C.D. Klaassen and M.O. Amdur, eds.), pp. 25-55, MacMillan, New York.

Kociba, R.J.,Keyes, D.G., Beyer, J.E., Carreon, R.M., Wade, C.E., Dittenber, D.A., Kalnins, R.P., Frauson, L.E., Park, C.N., Barnard, S.D., Hummel, R.A. and Humiston, C.G. (1978). Results of a two-year chronic toxicity and oncogenicity study of 2,3,7,8-tetrachlorodibenzo-p-dioxin in rats. *Toxicol. Appl. Pharmacol., 46*, 279-303.

Kodell, R.L., Farmer, J.A., Gaylor, D.W. and Cameron, A.M. (1982). Influence of cause-of-death assignment on time-to-tumor analyses in animal carcinogenesis studies. *J. Natl. Cancer Inst., 69*, 659-664.

Koizumi, A., Dobashi, Y., Tachibana, Y., Tsuda, K. and Katsunuma, H. (1974). Cytokinetic and cytogenetic changes in cultured human leukocytes and HeLa cells induced by benzene. *Ind. Health, 12*, 23-29.

Korczyn, A.D. and Eshel, Y. (1982). Mydriasis induced by tetrahydrocannabinol (THC) in rats. *Invest. Ophthalmol. Vis. Sci., 22*, 408-410.

Krasovskii, G.N. (1976). Extrapolation of experimental data from animals to man. *Environ. Health Perspect., 13*, 51.

Krewski, D., Clayson, D., Collins, B. and Munro, I.C. (1982). Toxicological procedures for assessing the carcinogenic potential of agricultural chemicals. In *Genetic Toxicology* (R.A. Fleck and A. Hollander, eds.), pp. 461-497, Plenum Press, New York.

Kriek, E. and Wetra, J.G. (1979). Metabolic activation of aromatic amines and amides and interactions with nucleic acids. In *Chemical Carcinogens and DNA* (P.L. Grover, ed.), pp.1-28, CRC Press, Boca Raton.

Kristofferson, U. (1972). Effect of cyclamate and saccharin on the chromosomes of a Chinese hamster cell line. *Hereditas, 70*, 271-282.

Kritzinger, E.E. and Bellhorn, R.W. (1982). Permeability of blood-retinal barriers in urethane-induced rat retinopathy: a fluorescein angiographic, vitreous fluorophotometric and fluorescence microscopic study. *Br. J. Ophthalmol., 66*, 630-635.

Kroes, R. (1979). Animal data, interpretation and consequences. In *Environmental Carcinogenesis* (P. Emmelot and E. Kriek, eds.), Elsevier/North Holland, Amsterdam.

Kroes, R. (1983). Short-term tests in the framework of carcinogen risk assessment to man. *Ann. N.Y. Acad. Sci., 407*, 398-408.

Kroes, R., Weiss, J.W. and Weisburger, J.H. (1975). Immunosuppression and chemical carcinogenesis: recent results. *Cancer Res., 52*, 65-75.

Krontiris, T.G. and Cooper, G.M. (1981). Transforming activity of human tumor DNAs. *Proc. Natl. Acad. Sci. U.S.A., 78*, 1181-1184.

Kubinski, H., Gutzke, G.E. and Kubinski, Z.O. (1981). DNA-cell-binding (DCB) assay for suspected carcinogens and mutagens. *Mutat. Res., 89*, 95-136.

Laerum, O.D. (1973). Reticulum cell neoplasms in normal and benzene treated hairless mice. *Acta Pathol. Microbiol. Scand., 81*, 57-63.

Lagakos, S. and Mosteller, F. (1981). A case study of statistics in the regulatory process: The FD&C Red No. 40 experiments. *J. Natl. Cancer Inst., 66*.

Lai, Y.L., Jacoby, R.O., Bhatt, P.N. and Jonas, A.M. (1976). Keratoconjunctivitis associated with sialodacryoadenitis in rats. *Invest. Ophthalmol., 15*(7), 538-541.

Lalwani, N.D., Reddy, M.K., Qureshi, S.A., Moehle, C.M.,Hayashi, H. and Reddy, J.K. (1983). Noninhibitory effect of antioxidant ethoxyquin 2(3)-tert-butyl-4-hyroxyanisole and 3,5,-di-tert-butyl-4-hydroxytoluene on hepatic peroxisome proliferation and peroxisomal fatty acid $\propto$-oxidation induced by a hypolipidemic agents in rats. *Cancer Res., 43*, 1680-1687.

Langmuir, I.S., Gottlieb, S.F., Pashko, L.L. and Martin, P. (1980). *In vivo* and *in vitro* induction of cytochrome P-450 synthesis in hyperexia. *Undersea Biomed. Res., 7*, 161.

Latt, S.A., Allen, J.W., Bloom, S.E., Carrano, A.V., Falke, E., Kram, D., Schneider, E.L., Schreck, R.R. and Tice, R.R. (1981). Sister-chromatid exchanges: a report of the Gene-Tox Program. *Mutat. Res., 87*, 17-62.

Lawson, A.T. and Hertzog, P. (1981). The failure of chronically administered saccharin to stimulate bladder epithelial DNA synthesis in F_0 rats. *Cancer Lett., 11*, 221-224.

Lebowitz, H., Brusick, D., Matheson, D., Reed, M., Goode, S. and Roy, G. (1978). The genetic activity of benzene in various short-term *in vitro* and *in vivo* assays for mutagenicity. *Proceedings of the Environmental Mutagens Society*, San Francisco, California.

Lee, K.P., Gibson, J.R., Sherman, H. (1979). Retinopathic effects of 2-aminooxypropionic acid derivatives in the rat. *Toxicol. Appl. Pharmacol., 51*, 219-232.

Legator, M.S. (1970a). Cited by S. S. Epstein in Staff Report for Nitrilotriacetic Acid (NTA) U.S. Senate Committee on Public Works.

Legator, M.S. (1970b). Cited by A.D. Little, Inc. Report: Status of environmental and human safety aspects of Nitrilotriacetic Acid (NTA), April, 1972

Legator, M.S. (1971). Cited by L.G. Scharpf, Jr. in Monsanto R&D report: Summary report on status of toxicological and environmental testing of Nitrilotriacetic Acid (NTA), August, 1974.

Legator, M.S. (1972). Chemical mutagens. *Ann. Rev. Med., 23*, 413-428.

Lessa, J.M.M., Becak, W., Rabello, M.N., Pereira, L.A.B. and Ungaro, M.T. (1976). Cytogenetic study of DDT on human lymphocytes *in vitro. Mutat. Res., 40*, 131-133.

Lethco, E.J. and Wallace, W.C., (1975). The metabolism of saccharin in animals. *Toxicology, 3*, 287-300.

Levin, W., Wood, A.W., Lu, A.V.H., Ryan, D. West, S., Conney, A.H., Thakker, D.R., Yagi, H. and Jerina, D.M. (1977). Role of purified cytochrome P-450 and epoxide hydrase in the activation and detoxification of benzo[a]pyrene. In *Drug Metabolism Concepts* (D.M. Jerina, ed.), pp. 99-126, American Chemical Society, Washington, D.C.

Lijinsky, W., Greenblatt, M. and Kommineni, C. (1973). Feeding studies of nitrilotriacetic acid and derivatives in rats. *J. Natl. Cancer Inst., 50*, 1061.

Lin, J.K., Miller, J.A. and Miller, E.C. (1977). 2,3-dihydro-2-(guan-7-yl)-3-hydroxy-aflatoxin B_1, a major acid hydrolysis product of aflatoxin B_1-DNA or -ribosomal RNA adducts formed in hepatic microsome-mediated reactions and in rat liver *in vivo. Cancer Res., 37*, 4430-4438.

Lindamood, C., Bedell, M.A., Billings, K.C., Dyroff, M.C. and Swenberg, J.A. (1984). Dose-response for DNA alkylation, [^{3}H] thymidine uptake into DNA, and 0-6-methylguanine-DNA methyltransferase activity in hepatocytes of rats and mice continuously exposed to dimethylnitrosamine. *Cancer Res.,44*, 196-200.

Litton Bionetics, Inc. (1973). Carcinogenicity of chemicals present in man's environment—final report. National Cancer Institute, January 31, 1973.

Litton Bionetics, Inc. (1978). Mutagenicity evaluation of sodium saccharin powder FCCX 17W 55585, Lot S-1648, Drum 40 and 41. Report submitted to Calorie Control Council, June 1978.

Loeb, L.A., Silber, J.R. and Fry, M. (1981). Infidelity of DNA replication in aging. In *Biological Mechanisms in Aging Conference Proceedings* (R.T. Schimke, ed.), pp. 270-278, NIH Publication # 81-2194.

Lohler, J. and Lehmann, G.F. (1979). Immunopathological alterations of lymphatic tissues in mice infected with lymphocytic choriomeningitis virus. *Adv. Exp. Med. Biol., 114*, 823-826.

Longacre, S.L., Kocsis, J.J. and Snyder, R. (1980). Benzene metabolism and toxicity in CD-1, C57/B6 and DBA/2N mice. In *Microsomes, Drug Oxidations and Chemical Carcinogenesis* (M.J. Coon, A. Conney, R.W. Estabrook, H.V. Gelboin, J.R. Gillette and P.J. O'Brien, eds.), pp. 897-902, Academic Press, New York.

Longacre, S.L., Kocsis, J.J. and Snyder, R. (1981a). Toxicological and biochemical effects of repeated administration of benzene in mice. *Toxicol. Environ. Health, 7*, 223-237.

Longacre, S.L., Kocsis, J.J., Witmer, C.M., Lee, E.W., Sammett, D. and Snyder, R. (1981b). Influence of strain differences in mice on the metabolism and toxicity of benzene. *Toxicol. Appl. Pharmacol., 60*, 398-409.

Loprieno, N. (1980). Evaluation and relevance of yeast and molds in the screening tests for carcinogenicity. In *The Predictive Value of In Vitro Short-Term Screening Tests in Carcinogenicity Evaluation* (G.M. Williams, R. Kroes, H.W. Waaijers and K.W. van de Poll, eds.), Elsevier/North Holland, Amsterdam.

Lundy, J., Lovett, E.J. and Conran, P. (1977). Pulmonary metastases, a potential biologic consequence of anesthetic-induced immunosuppression by thiopental. *Surgery, 82*, 254-256.

Lüning, K.G. (1970). Cited by S. S. Epstein in Staff Report for NTA to U.S. Senate Committee on Public Works.

Lüning, K.G. *et al.* (1970). Cited by S.S. Epstein in *Int. J. Environ. Studies, 2*, 291 (1972).

Lutz, W. (1979). *In vivo* covalent binding of organic chemicals to DNA as a quantitative indicator in the process of chemical carcinogenesis. *Mutat. Res., 65*, 289-356.

Lutz, W.K. and Schlatter, C.H. (1977). Saccharin does not bind to DNA of liver or bladder of the rat. *Chem.-Biol. Interact., 19*, 253-257.

Madhaven, T.V. and Gopalan, C. (1968). The effect of dietary protein on carcinogenesis of aflatoxin. *Arch. Pathol., 85*, 133-137.

Madhukar, B.V. and Matsumura, F. (1979). Comparison of induction patterns of rat hepatic microsomal mixed-function oxidases by pesticides and related chemicals. *Pestic. Biochem. Physiol., 11*, 301-308.

Magee, P.N., Montesano, R. and Preussmann, R. (1976). N-Nitroso compounds and related carcinogens. In *Chemical Carcinogens* (C.E. Searle, ed.), pp. 491-625, American Chemical Society, Washington, D.C.

Manara, L., Coccia, P. and Croci, T. (1982). Persistent tissue levels of TCDD in the mouse and their reduction as related to prevention of toxicity. *Drug Metab. Rev., 13*, 423-446.

Manara, L., Cerlette, C. and Mennine, T. (1976). Prevention by calcium administration of reserpine action on rat brain noradrenalin stores: a reappraisal. *Res. Commun. Chem. Pathol. Pharmacol., 14*, 471-487.

Manara, L. and Garattini, S. (1967). Time course of ^{3}H- reserpine levels in brains of normal and tetrabenazine-pretreated rats. *Eur. J. Pharmacol., 2*, 139.

Mantel, N. (1980). Assessing laboratory evidence for neoplastic activity. *Biometrics, 36*, 389-399.

Marshall, E. (1982). EPA's high risk carcinogen policy. *Science, 218*, 957-958. (See also related letter: Todhunter, J.A. and Weinstein, I.B. *Science, 219*, 795-796.)

Marshall, T.C., Dorough, H.W. and Swim, H.E. (1976). Screening of pesticides for mutagenic potential using *Salmonella typhimurium* mutants. *J. Agric. Food Chem., 24*, 560-563.

Martin, C.N., McDermid, A.C. and Garner, R.C. (1978). Testing of known carcinogens and non-carcinogens for their ability to induce unscheduled DNA-synthesis in HeLa cells. *Cancer Res., 38*, 2621-2627.

Marx, J.L. (1982). Cancer cell genes linked to oncogenes. *Science, 216*, 724.

Maslansky, C.J. and Williams, G.M. (1981). Evidence for an epigenetic mode of action on organochlorine pesticide hepatocarcinogenicity: a lack of genotoxicity in rat, mouse and hamster hepatocytes. *J. Toxicol. Environ. Health, 8*, 121-130.

Mason, J.M., Green, M.M., Shaw, K.E. and Boyd, J.B. (1981). Genetic analysis of X-linked mutagen-sensitive mutants of *Drosophila melanogaster. Mutat. Res., 81*, 329-343.

Masubuchi, M., Yoshida, S., Hiraga, K. and Nawai, S. (1978). The mutagenicity of sodium saccharin. II. Cytogenetic studies (Abstract). *Mutat. Res., 54*, 219.

McCann, J.C. (1977). *Cancer Testing Technology and Saccharin, Appendix II, Short-term Tests*. Office of Technology Assessment, Congress of the United States, pp. 91-143.

McCann, J. and Ames, B.N. (1976). Detection of carcinogens as mutagens in the *Salmonella*/microsome tests: assay of 300 chemicals. *Proc. Natl. Acad. Sci., U.S.A., 73*, 950-954.

McCann, J., Choi, E., Yamasaki, E. and Ames, B.N. (1975). Detection of carcinogens as mutagens in the *Salmonella*/microsome test: assay of 300 chemicals. *Proc. Natl. Acad. Sci., U.S.A., 72*, 5135-5139.

Melnick, R.L., Boorman, G.A., Haseman, J.K., Montali, R.J. and Huff, J. (1984). Urolithiasis and bladder carcinogenicity of melamine in rodents. *Toxicol. Appl. Pharmacol., 72*, 292-303.

Meltzer, M.S. (1976). Tumoricidal responses *in vitro* of peritoneal macrophages from conventionally housed and germ-free nude mice. *Cell Immunol.,22*, 176-181.

Michael, W.R. and Wakim, J.M. (1971). Metabolism of nitrilotriacetic acid (NTA). *Toxicol. Appl. Pharmacol., 18*, 407.

Miller, A.B. and Howe, G.R. (1977). Artificial sweeteners and human bladder cancer. *Lancet, 2*, 578-581.

Miller, C.L. and Claudy, B.J. (1979). Suppressor T-cell activity induced as a result of thermal injury. *Cell Immunol., 44*, 201-208.

Miller, C.T., Neutel, C.I., Nair, R.C., Marrett, L.D., Last, J.M. and Collins, W.E. (1978). Relative importance of risk factors in bladder carcinogenesis. *J. Chronic Dis., 1*, 51-56.

Miller, E. (1978). Some current perspectives on chemical carcinogenesis in humans and experimental animals: Presidential Address. *Cancer Res., 38*, 1479-1496.

Miller, E.C. and Miller, J.A. (1976). The metabolism of chemical carcinogens to reactive electrophiles and their possible mechanism of action in carcinogenesis. In *Chemical Carcinogens* (C.E. Searle, ed.), pp. 737-762, American Chemical Society, Washington, D.C.

Miller, E.C., Miller, J.A. and Enomoto, M. (1964). The comparative carcinogenicities of 2-acetyl-aminofluorene and its N-metabolite, hydroxy, in mice, hamsters and guinea pigs. *Cancer Res., 24*, 2018-2032.

Miller, J.A. (1970). Carcinogenesis by chemicals—an overview. G.H.A. Clowes Memorial Lecture, *Cancer Res.*, 30, 559-576.

Miller, J.A. and Miller, E.C. (1969). Physiochemical mechanisms of carcinogenicity. In *Jerusalem Symposium on Quantum Chemistry and Biochemistry* (E.D. Bergmann and B. Pullman, eds.), pp. 237-261, Israel Academy of Sciences and Humanities, Jerusalem.

Minegishi, I.I., Asahima, M. and Yamaha, T. (1972). The metabolism of saccharin and related compounds in rats and guinea pigs. *Chem. Pharmacol. Bull., 20*, 1351.

Mitchell, J.R., Potter, D.J., Davis, W.Z., Gillette, J.R. and Brodie, B.B. (1973). Acetaminophen-induced hepatic necrosis. I. Role of metabolism, *J. Pharmacol. Exp. Ther., 187*, 185.

Mizutani, T. and Mitsuoka, T. (1979). Effect of intestinal bacteria on incidence of liver tumors in gnotobiotic C3H/He male mice. *J. Natl. Cancer Inst., 63*, 1365-1370.

Mollet, P. (1975). Toxicity and mutagenicity of ethylenethiourea (ETU) in *Drosophila. Mutat. Res., 29*, 254.

Mondal, S., Brankow, D.W. and Heidelberger, C. (1978). Enhancement of oncogenesis in $C_3H/10T$-1/2 mouse embryo cell culture by saccharin. *Science, 201*, 1141-1142.

Montesano, R., Rajewsky, M.F., Pegg, A.E., and Miller, E. (1982). Development and possible use of immunological techniques to detect individual exposure to carcinogens. International Agency for Research on Cancer/International Programme on Chemical Safety Working Group Report. *Cancer Res., 42*, 5236-5239.

Moore, C.W. and A. Schmick (1979). Genetic effects of impure and pure saccharin in yeast. *Science, 205*, 1007-1010.

Morgan, R.W. and Jain, M.S. (1974). Bladder cancer: smoking, beverages, and artificial sweeteners. *J. Chronic Dis., 111*, 1067-1070.

Morgan, D.P. and Roan, C.C. (1971). Absorption, storage and metabolic conversion of ingested DDT and DDT metabolites in man. *Arch. Environ. Health, 22*, 301-308.

Mori, T., Nagasawa, H. and Bern, H.A. (1980). Long-term effects of perinatal exposure to hormones on normal and neoplastic mammary growth in rodents: a review. *J. Environ. Pathol. Toxicol., 3*, 191-205.

Morimoto, K. (1976). Analysis of combined effects of benzene with radiation on chromosomes in cultured human leukocytes. *Jpn. J. Ind. Health (Sangyo Igaku), 18*, 23-24.

Morimoto, K. and Wolff, S. (1980). Increase of sister chromatid exchanges and perturbations of cell division kinetics in human lymphocytes by benzene metabolites. *Cancer Res., 40*, 1189-1193.

Morrison, A.S. and Buring, J.E. (1980). Artificial sweeteners and cancer of the lower urinary tract. *New Engl. J. Med., 302*, 537-541.

Moslen, M.T., Reynolds, E.S. and Szabo, S. (1977). Enhancement of the metabolism and hepatotoxicity of trichloroethylene and perchloroethylene. *Biochem. Pharmacol., 26*, 369-375.

Munro, I.C. (1977). Considerations in chronic toxicity testing: the chemical, the dose, the design. *J. Environ. Pathol. Toxicol., 1*, 183-197.

Munro, I.C., Moodie, C.A., Krewski, D. and Grice H.C. (1975). Carcinogenicity study of commercial saccharin in the rat. *Toxicol. Appl. Pharmacol. 32*, 513-526.

Münzer, M. and Heder, K. (1972). Results of industrial-medical and technical examination of chemical purification operations. *Zbl. Arbeitsmed., 22*, 133-138.

Murasaki, G. and Cohen, S.M. (1981). Effect of dose of sodium saccharin on the induction of rat urinary bladder proliferation. *Cancer Res., 41*, 942-944.

Murphy, S.D. (1980). Assessment of the potential for toxic interactions among environmental pollutants. In *The Principles and Methods in Modern Toxicology* (C.L. Galli, S.D. Murphy and R. Paoletti, eds.), pp. 277-294, Elsevier/North Holland, Amsterdam.

Murray, A.W. and Fitzgerald, D.J. (1979). Tumor promoters inhibit metabolic cooperation in co-cultures of epidermal and 3T3 cells. *Biochem. Biophys. Res. Commun., 91*, 393.

Napalkov, N.P. (1976). Tumors of the thyroid gland. In *Pathology of Tumors in Laboratory Animals, Vol.I., Tumors of the Rat, Part 2.* (V.S. Turusov, ed.), pp. 239-271, International Agency for Research on Cancer, Lyon.

Natarajan, A.T. and Obe, G. (1982). Mutagenicity testing with cultured mammalian cells: cytogenetic assays. In *Mutagenicity, New Horizons in Genetic Toxicology* (J.A Heddle, ed.), pp. 172-213, Academic Press, New York.

NAS (National Academy of Sciences) (1975). *Principles for Evaluation of Chemicals in the Environment.* p. 118, National Academy Press, Washington, D.C.

NAS (National Academy of Sciences) (1979). *Saccharin: Technical Assessment of Risks and Benefits*. Committee for a study on saccharin and food safety policy, Report No. 1, National Academy Press, Washington, D.C.

NAS (National Academy of Sciences) (1980). *Principles of Toxicological Interactions Associated with Multiple Chemical Exposures*. National Academy Press, Washington, D.C.

NCI (National Cancer Institute) (1976). Carcinogenesis bioassay of chloroform. *National Technical Information Service*, No. PB264018/AS (March).

NCI (National Cancer Institute) (1977a). Bioassay of chlordane for possible carcinogenicity. *Technical Report Series*, No. 8.

NCI (National Cancer Institute) (1977b). Bioassays of nitrilotriacetic acid (NTA) and nitrilotriacetic acid, trisodium salt, monohydrate ($Na_3NTA.H_2O$) for possible carcinogenicity (NCI-CG-TR-6). *DHEW Publication No.* (NIH) 77-806.

NCI (National Cancer Institute) (1980a). Bioassay of 2,3,7,8-tetrachlorodibenzo-p-dioxin (gavage study). *DHHS Publication No.* (NIH) 80-1765. Carcinogenesis testing program, National Cancer Institute, National Institutes of Health, Bethesda.

NCI (National Cancer Institute) (1980b). Bioassay of 2,3,7,8-tetrachlorodibenzo-p-dioxin for possible carcinogenicity. Technical Report No. 201, *DHHS Publication No.* (NIH) 80-1757. U.S. Department of Health and Human Services, Public Health Service, National Institutes of Health, Bethesda.

National Toxicology Program Technical Report (1983). *Carcinogenesis Bioassay of Melamine*. Technical Report No. 245, *DHHS Publication No.* (NIH) 83-2501. Washington, D.C.

Nebert, D.W., Thorgeirsson, S.S. and Felton, J.S. (1976). Genetic differences in mutagenesis, carcinogenesis and drug toxicity. In *In Vitro Metabolic Activation in Mutagenesis Testing* (F.J. de Serres, J.R. Fouts, J.R. Bend and R.M. Philpot, eds.), pp. 105-124, Elsevier/North Holland, Amsterdam.

Neukomm, S. (1962). Co-carcinogenic action of various fractions of tobacco smoke. *Acta Unio Int. Cancrum, 18*, 33-36.

Newberry, B.H. (1981). Effects of presumably stressful stimulation (PSS) on the development of animal tumors: some issues. In *Perspectives on Behavioral Medicine* (S.M. Weiss, J.A. Herd and B.H. Fox, eds.), Proceedings of the Academy of Behavioral Medicine Research Conference, pp. 329-349, Academic Press, New York.

Newell, G.W., and Maxwell W.A. (1972). Study of mutagenic effects of saccharin (insoluble), XPBRC #221824/6, U.S. Government Report.

Newell, G.R., Hoover, R.N. and Kolbye, A.C. (1978). Status report on saccharin in humans. *J. Natl. Cancer Inst., 61*, 275-276.

Nixon, G.A., Buehler, E.V. and Niewenhuis, R.J. (1972). Two-year rat feeding study with trisodium nitrilotriacetate and its calcium chelate. *Toxicol. Appl. Pharmacol., 21*, 244.

Nishizumi, M. (1979). Effect of phenobarbital, dichlorodiphenyl trichloroethane and polychlorinated biphenyls on diethylnitrosamine-induced hepatocarcinogenesis. *Gann, 70*, 835-837.

Noell, W.K. and Albrecht, R. (1971). Irreversible effects of visible light on the retina: the role of vitamin A. *Science, 172*, 76-80.

Noell, W.K., Walker, V.S., Kans, B.S. and Berman, S. (1966). Retinal damage by light in rats. *Invest. Ophthalmol., 5*, 450-473.

Nutrition Foundation (1983). *The Relevance of Mouse Liver Hepatoma to Human Carcinogenic Risk.* A report of the International Expert Advisory Committee to the Nutrition Foundation, pp. 1-34, Washington, D.C.

Nylander, P.O., Olofsson, H., Rasmuson, B. and Svahlin, J. (1978). Mutagenic effects of petrol in *Drosophila melanogaster*. I. Effects of benzene and 1,2-dichloroethane. *Mutat. Res., 57*, 163-167.

Ochi, H., and Tonomura, A. (1978). Presence of unscheduled DNA synthesis in cultured human cells after treatment with sodium saccharin. *Mutat. Res.* (Abstract), *54*, 224.

Ogata, M., Takatsuka, Y. and Tomokuni, K. (1971). Excretion of organic chlorine compounds in the urine of persons exposed to vapors of trichloroethylene and tetrachloroethylene. *Br. J. Ind. Med., 28*, 386-391.

Okita, K. (1976). Cytochrome P-450 in hyperplastic liver nodules during hepatocarcinogenesis with C-2- fluorenyl- acetamide in rats. *Gann, 67*, 899-902.

O'Neil, T.P., Brimer, T.P., Machanoff, R., Hirsch, G.P. and Hsie, A.W. (1977). A quantitative assay of mutation induction at the hypoxanthine-guanine phosphoribosyltransferase locus in Chinese hamster ovary cells (CHO/HGPRT system): development and definition of the system. *Mutat. Res., 45*, 95-101.

OECD (Organization of Economic and Cooperative Development) (1981). *Test Guidelines for Carcinogenicity Studies.* OECD Long-term Expert Group.

O'Steen, W.K., Anderson, K.V. and Shear, C.R. (1974). Photoreceptor degeneration in albino rats: dependency on age. *Invest. Ophthalmol., 13*, 334-339.

Ott, G. (1970). *Frendkörpersorkome Experimentelle Medizin, Patholgie und Klinik,* Volume 32, Springer Verlag, Berlin.

Pacifici, G.M., Boobis, A.R., Brodie, M.J., McManus, M.E. and Davies, D.S. (1981). Tissue and species differences in enzymes of epoxide metabolism. *Xenobiotica, 11*, 73-79.

Page, N.P. (1977). Concepts of a bioassay program in environmental carcinogens. In *Advances in Modern Toxicology, Vol. 3, Environmental Cancer* (H.F. Kraybill and M.A. Mehlman, eds.), pp. 87-171, John Wiley, New York.

Paika, J., Beauchesne, M., Randall, M., Schreck, R. and Nate, S. (1981). *In vivo* SCE analysis of 20 coded compounds. In *Evaluation of Short-Term Tests for Carcinogens* (F.J. de Serres and J. Ashby, eds.), Elsevier/North Holland, New York.

Palmer, A.K., Street, A.E., Roe, F.J.C., Worden, A.N. and van Abbé, N. (1979). Safety evaluation of toothpaste containing chloroform. II. Long-term studies in rats. *J. Environ. Pathol. Toxicol., 2*, 821-833.

Pani, P., Porcu, M., Columbano, A., Dessi, S., Ledda, G.M. and Diaz, G. (1978). Differential effects of choline administration on liver microsomes of female and male rats. *Exp. Mol. Pathol., 28*, 154.

Parke, D.V. (1981a). The endoplasmic reticulum: its role in physiological functions and pathological situations. In *Concepts in Drug Metabolism,* Part B, (P. Jenner and B. Testa, eds.), pp. 1-52, Marcel Dekker, New York.

Parke, D.V. (1981b). Cytochrome P-450 and the detoxification of environmental chemicals. *Aquatic Toxicol., 1*, 367.

Parke, D.V. (1982). The disposition and metabolism of environmental chemicals by mammalia. In *The Handbook of Environmental Chemistry* Volume 2: Section B, *Reaction and Processes* (O. Hutzinger, ed.), pp. 141-178, Springer/Verlag, Berlin.

Parke, D.V. and Ioannides, C. (1981a). Role of mixed function oxidases in the formation of biological intermediates. *Adv. Exp. Med. Biol., 136*, 23.

Parke, D.V. and Ioannides, C. (1981b). The role of nutrition in toxicology. *Ann. Rev. Nutr., 1*, 207-234.

Parke, D.V. and Williams, R.T. (1953). Studies in detoxification. The metabolism of benzene containing *14C- benzene. Biochem. J., 54*, 231-238.

Parker, J.C., Bahlman, L.J., Leidel, N.A., Stein, H.P., Thomas, A.W., Wolf, B.S. and Baier, E.J. (1978). Current NIOSH intelligence Bulletin No. 20: Tetrachloroethylene (perchloroethylene). *Am. Ind. Hyg. Assoc. J., 39*, 13 A23-A29.

Parker, J.C. and Richter, C.B. (1982). Viral diseases of the respiratory system. In *The Mouse in Biomedical Research, Volume II. Diseases* (H.L. Foster, J.D. Small and J.G. Fox, eds.), p. 122, Academic Press, New York.

Parry, J.M., Parry, E.M. and Barrett, P.C. (1981). Tumor promoters induce mitotic aneuploidy in yeast. *Nature, 294*, 263-265.

Pegg, A.E. and Hui, G. (1978). Formation and subsequent removal of 6-methyl-guanine from deoxyribonucleic acid in rat liver and kidney after small doses of dimethylnitrosamine. *Biochem. J., 173*, 739-748.

Pegg, D.G., Zempel, J.A., Braun, W.H. and Watanabe, P.G. (1979). Disposition of tetrachloro-(^{14}C)-ethylene following oral and inhalation exposures in rats. *Toxicol. Appl. Pharmacol., 51*, 465-474.

Peraino, C., Fry, R.J.M., Stoffeldt, E. and Christopher, J.P. (1975). Comparative enhancing effects of phenobarbital, amobarbitol, diphenylhydantoin and dichlorodiphenyltrichloroethane or 2-acetylaminofluorine-induced hepatic tumorigenesis in the rat. *Cancer Res., 35*, 2884-2890.

Peraino C., Staffeldt, E.F., Haugen, D.A., Lombard, L.S., Stevens, F.J. and Fry, R.J.M. (1980). Effects of varying the dietary concentration of phenobarbital on its enhancement of 2-acetylaminofluorine-induced hepatic tumorigenesis. *Cancer Res., 40*, 3268-3273.

Peterson, J.E. and Robinson, W.H. (1964). Metabolic products of p,p'DDT in the rat. *Toxicol. Appl. Pharmacol., 6*, 321-327.

Peto, R., Pike, M.C., Day, N.E., Gray, R.G., Lee, P.N., Parish, S., Peto, J., Richards, S. and Wahrendorf, J. (1980). Guidelines for simple, sensitive significance tests for carcinogenic effects in long-term animal experiments. In *Long-term and Short-term Screening Assays for Carcinogens: A Critical Appraisal.* IARC Monographs on the Evaluations of the Carcinogenic Risk of Chemicals to Humans, Annex to Supplement 2, pp. 311-426, International Agency for Research on Cancer, Lyon.

Pienta, R.J., Poiley, T.A. and Lebherz, W.B. (1977). Morphological transformation of early passage golden Syrian hamster embryo cells derived from cryopreserved primary cultures as a reliable *in vitro* bioassay for identifying diverse carcinogens. *Int. J. Cancer, 19*, 642-655.

Pienta, R.J. (1980). Evaluation and relevance of the Syrian hamster embryo cell system. In *The Predictive Value of In Vitro Short-Term Screening Tests in Carcinogenicity Evaluation* (G.M. Williams, R. Kroes, H.W. Waaijers and K.W. van de Poll, eds.), pp. 149-169, Elsevier/North Holland, Amsterdam.

Pinder, R.M., Brogden, R.N., Sawyer, P.R., Speight, T.M., Spencer, R. and Avery, G.S. (1976). Carbenoxolone: a review of its pharmacological properties and therapeutic efficacy in peptic ulcer disease. *Drugs, 11*, 245.

Pitkin, R.M., Anderson, D.W., Reynolds, W.A. and Filer, L.J. (1971). Saccharin metabolism in *Macacca mulatta*. *Proc. Soc. Exp. Biol. Med. U.S.A., 137*, 803.

Pitot, H.C., Goldsworthy, T., Campbell, H.A. and Poland, A. (1980). Quantitative evaluation of the promotion by 2,3,7,8-tetrachlorodibenzo-p-dioxin of hepatocarcinogenesis from diethylnitrosamine. *Cancer Res., 40*, 3616-3620.

Pitot, H.C. and Sirica, A.E. (1980). The stages of initiation and promotion in hepatocarcinogenesis. *Biochim. Biophys. Acta, 605*, 191-215.

Planche, G., Croisy, A., Malaveille, C., Tomatis, L. and Bartsch, H.(1979). Metabolic and mutagenicity studies on DDT and 15 derivatives. Detection of 1,1-bis(p-chlorophenyl)-2,2-dichloroethane and 1,1-bis(p-chlorophenyl)-2,2,2-trichloro- ethyl acetate (kelthane acetate) as mutagenic in *Salmonella typhimurium* and of 1,1-bis(p-chlorophenyl)ethylene oxide, a likely metabolite, as an alkylating agent. *Chem.-Biol. Interact., 25*, 157-175.

Pletscher, A. and Besendorf, H. (1959). Antagonism between hormaline and long-acting monoamine oxidase inhibitors concerning the effect on 5-hydroxytryptamine and norepinephrine metabolism in the brain. *Experientia, 15*, 25.

Pohl, L. (1979). Biochemical toxicology of chloroform. In *Reviews in Biochemical Toxicology* (E. Hodgson, J.R. Bend and R.M. Philpot, eds.), pp. 79-107, Elsevier/North Holland, New York.

Pohl, L.R., Bhooshan, B., Whittaker, N.F. and Krishna, G. (1977). Phosgene: a potential metabolite of chloroform. *Biochem. Biophys. Res. Commun., 79*, 684-691.

Poland, A. and Glover, E. (1979). An estimate of the maximum *in vivo* covalent binding the 2,3,7,8-tetrachlorodibenzo-p-dioxin to rat liver protein, ribosomal RNA and DNA. *Cancer Res., 39*, 3341-3344.

Poland, A., and Kende, A.S. (1976). 2,3,7,8-tetrachlorodibenzo-p-dioxin: environmental contaminant and molecular probe. *Fed. Proc. 35*, 2404-2411.

Pooke, T. and Parke, D. (1978). Effect of age inducing agents and carcinogens on the distribution of cytochrome P-450 in microsomal membranes from rat liver. *Biochem. Soc. Trans., 6*, 959-961.

Pool, B. (1978). Non-mutagenicity of saccharin. *Toxicology, 11*, 95-97.

Potter, W.Z., Thorgeirsson, S.S., Jollow, D.J. and Mitchell, J.R., (1974). Acetaminophen-induced hepatic necrosis. V. Correlation of hepatic necrosis, covalent binding and glutathione depletion in hamsters. *Pharmacology, 12*, 129.

Pound, G.W. (1974). Internal report, Monsanto Chemical Corporation.

Prehn, R.T. (1973). Destruction of tumor as an "innocent bystander"in an immune response specifically directed against nontumor antigens. *Is. J. Med. Sci., 9*, 375-379.

Preston, R.J., Au, W., Bender, M.A., Brewer, J.G., Carrano, A.V., Heddle, J.A., McFee, A.F., Wolff, S. and Wassom, J.S. (1981). Mammalian *in vivo* and *in vitro* cytogenetic assays. A report of the U.S. EPA Gene-Tox program. *Mutat. Res., 87*, 143-188.

Price, N.R. (1975). The effect of two insecticides on the $Ca^{+2}+Mg^{+2}$-activated ATPase of the sarcoplasmic reticulum on the flounder, *Platichthys flesus. Comp. Biochem. Physiol., 55C*, 91-94.

Price, P.J., Hassett, C.M. and Mansfield, J.I. (1978). Transforming potential of trichloro-ethylene and proposed industrial alternatives. *In Vitro, 14*, 290-293.

Probst, G.S., McMahon, R.E., Hill, L.E., Thompson, C.Z., Epp, J.K. and Neal, S.B. (1981). Chemically-induced unscheduled DNA synthesis in primary rat hepatocyte cultures: a comparison with bacterial mutagenicity using 218 compounds. *Environ. Mutat., 3*, 11-32.

Puccetti, P., Santoni, A. Riccardi, C. and Herberman, R.B. (1980). Cytotoxic effector cells with the characteristics of natural killer cells in the lungs of mice. *Int. J. Cancer, 75*, 153-158.

Purchase, I.F.H. (1980). Inter-species comparisons of carcinogenicity. *Br. J. Cancer, 41*, 454-468.

Purchase, I.F.H. (1982). An appraisal of predictive tests for carcinogenicity. *Mutat. Res., 99*, 53.

Quinn, G.P., Axelrod, J. and Brodie, B.B. (1958). Species strain and sex differences in metabolism of hexobarbitone, amidopyrine, antipyrine and aniline. *Biochem. Pharmacol., 1*, 152.

Radman, M., Villani, G., Boiteux, S., Defais, M., Caillet-Fauquet, P. and Spadari, S. (1977). On the mechanism and genetic control of mutagenesis induced by carcinogenic mutagens. In *Origins of Human Cancer* (H.H. Hiatt, J.D. Watson and J.A. Winsten, eds.), pp. 903-922, Cold Spring Harbor Laboratory, New York.

Radzialowski, F.M. and Bousquet, W.F. (1968). Daily rhythmic variation in hepatic drug metabolism in the rat and mouse. *J. Pharmacol. Exp. Ther., 163*, 229-238.

Rall, D.P. (1977a). Species differences in carcinogenicity testing. In *Origins of Human Cancer* (H.H. Hiatt, J.D. Watson and J.A. Winsten, eds.), pp. 1383-1390, Cold Spring Harbor Laboratory, New York.

Rall, D.P. (1977b). The role of laboratory animal studies in estimating carcinogenic risks in man. In *Carcinogenic Risks—Strategies for Intervention* (W. Davis and C. Rosenfeld, eds.), IARC Scientific Publications, Lyon.

Rampy, L.W., Quast, J.F., Leong, B.K.J. and Gehring, P.J.(1977). Results of long term inhalation toxicity studies on rats of 1,1,1-trichloroethane and perchloroethylene formula-tions (Abstract). In *International Congress on Toxicology, 27*, Toronto, Canada.

Ramsey, J.C. and Reitz, R.H. (1981). Pharmacokinetics and threshold concepts. *Am. Chem. Soc. Symp. Ser., 160*, 239.

Rasmussen, R.E. (1980). Repair of chemical carcinogen-induced lesions. In *Genetic Differences in Chemical Carcinogenesis* (R.E. Kouri, ed.), pp. 67-99, CRC Press, Boca Raton.

Razin, A. and Friedman, J. (1981). DNA methylation and its possible biological roles. *Prog. Nucleic Acid Res. Mol. Biol., 25*, 33-52.

Reddy, B.S., Weisburger, J.H., Wynder, E.L. (1978). Colon cancer: bile salts as tumor promoters. In *Mechanisms of Tumor Promotion and Cocarcinogenesis* (T.J. Slaga, R.K. Boutwell and A. Sivak, eds.), Vol. 2, pp. 453-464, Raven Press, New York.

Reddy, E.P., Reynolds, R.K., Santos, E., and Barbacid, M. (1982a). A point mutation is responsible for the acquistion of transforming properties by the T24 human bladder carcinoma oncogene. *Nature* (London), *300*, 149-152.

Reddy, J.K., Azarnoff, D.L. and Hignite, C.E. (1980). Hypolipidemic hepatic peroxisome proliferators form a novel class of chemical carcinogens. *Nature* (London), *283*, 397-398.

Reddy, J.K., Lalwani, N.D., Reddy, M.K., and Qureshi, S.A. (1982b). Excessive accumulation of autofluorescent lipofuscin in the liver during hepatocarcinogenesis by methyl clofenapate and other hypolipidemic peroxisome proliferators. *Cancer Res., 42*, 259-266.

Reddy, J.K. and Qureshi, S.A. (1979). Tumorigenicity of the hypolipidemic peroxisome proliferator ethyl-p-chlorophenoxyisobutyrate (clofibrate) in rats. *Br. J. Cancer, 40*, 476.

Reddy, J.K. and Rao, M.S. (1977). Development of liver tumors in rats treated with the peroxisomal enzyme inducer nafenopin. *Am. J. Pathol., 86*, 2.

Reeves, P.R., Barnfield, D.J., Langshaw, S., McIntosh, D.A.D. and Winrow, M.J. (1978). Disposition and metabolism of atenolol in animals. *Xenobiotica, 8*, 305.

Reiter, R.J. and Klein, D.C. (1971). Observations on the pineal gland, the harderian glands, the retina and the reproductive organs of adult female rats exposed to continuous light. *J. Endocr., 51*, 117-125.

Reitz, R.H., Gehring, P.J. and Park, C.N. (1978). Carcinogenic risk estimation for chloroform: an alternative to EPA's procedures. *Food Cosmet. Toxicol., 16*, 511-514.

Reitz, R.H., Quast, J.F., Stott, W.T., Watanabe, P.G. and Gehring, P.J. (1980a). Pharmacokinetics and macromolecular effects of chloroform in rats and mice: implications for carcinogenic risk estimation. In *Water Chlorination: Environmental Impact and Health Effects* (R.L. Jolley, W.A. Brungs and R.B. Cumming, eds.), Vol. 3, pp. 983-993, Ann Arbor Science Publishers, Ann Arbor.

Reitz, R.H., Watanabe, P.G., McKenna, M.J., Quast, J.E. and Gehring, P.J. (1980b). Effects of vinylidene chloride on DNA synthesis and DNA repair in the rat and mouse: a comparative study with dimethylnitrosamine. *Toxicol. Appl. Pharmacol., 52*, 357-370.

Remmer, H. (1969). The induction of hydroxylating enzymes by drugs. In *Biomedical Aspects of Antimetabolites and Drug Hydroxylation*, Federation of European Biological Societies Symposium (D. Shugar, ed.), p. 125, Academic Press, London.

Renwick, A.G. (1981). The fate of saccharin in rat and man; species and dose considerations. Environmental Medicine Symposium: *An Academic Review of the Safety Assessment of Artificial Sweeteners*. May 13, 1981.

Renwick, A.G. and Sweatman, T.W. (1979). The absorption of saccharin from the rat urinary bladder. *J. Pharm. Pharmacol., 31*, 650-652.

Renwick, A.G. and Williams, R.T. (1978). The saccharin story, another installment. *Food Cosmet. Toxicol.*, 16.

Reznikoff, C.A., Bertram, J.S., Brankow, D.W. and Heidelberger, C. (1973). Quantitative and qualitative studies of chemical transformation of cloned C3H mouse embryo cells sensitive to postconfluence inhibition of division. *Cancer Res.*, *33*, 3239-3249.

Riccardi, C., Puccetii, P., Santoni, A. and Berberman, R.B. (1979). Rapid *in vivoassay of mouse natural killer cell activity. J. Natl. Cancer Inst.*, *63*, 1041-1045.

Riccardi, C., Santoni, A., Barlozzari, T., Puccetti, P. and Herberman, R.B. (1980). *In vivo* natural reactivity of mice against tumor cells. *Int. J. Cancer, 255*, 475-486.

Rickert, D.E., Baker, T.S., Bus, J.S., Barrow, C.S. and Irons, R.D. (1979). Benzene disposition in the rat after exposure by inhalation. *Toxicol. Appl. Pharmacol., 49*, 417-423.

Riley, V. (1975). Mouse mammary tumors: alterations of incidence as apparent functions of stress. *Science, 189*, 465-467.

Riley, V. (1981). Psychoneuroendocrine influences on immunocompetence and neoplasia. *Science, 212*, 1100-1109.

Riley, V., Spackman, D.H., Santisteban, G.A., Dalldorf, G., Hellstrom, I., Hellstrom, K.-E., Lance, E.M., Rowson, K.E.K., Mahy, B.W.J., Alexander, P., Stock, C.C., Sjogren, H.O., Hollander, V.P. and Horzinek, M.C. (1978). The LDH virus: an interfering biological contaminant (letter). *Science, 200*, 124-126.

Rinkus, S.J., and Legator, M.S. (1979). Chemical characterization of 465 known or suspected carcinogens and their correlation with mutagenic activity in the *Salmonella typhimuriumsystem. Cancer Res.*, *39*, 3289-3318.

Rizzino, A., Gonda, M.A. and Rapp. U.R. (1982). Dome formation by a retrovirus-induced lung adenocarcinoma cell line. *Cancer Res., 42(5)*, 1881-1887.

Robison, W.G. and Kuwabara, T. (1976). Light-induced alterations in retinal pigment epithelium in black, albino and beige mice. *Exp. Eye Res., 22*, 549-557.

Roe, F.J.C., Bosch, D. and Boutwell, R.K. (1958). The carcinogenicity of creosote oil: the induction of skin tumors in mice. *Cancer Res., 18*, 1171-1175.

Roe, F.J.C., Palmer, A.K., Worden, W.N. and van Abbé (1979). Safety evaluation of toothpaste containing chloroform. I. Long-term studies in mice. *J. Environ. Pathol. Toxicol., 2*, 799-819.

Rogers A.E. (1975). Variable effects of a lipotrope deficient high-fat diet on chemical carcinogenesis in rats. *Cancer Res., 35*, 2469-2474.

Rogers, A.E.(1983). Influence of dietary content of lipids and lipotropic nutrients on chemical carcinogenesis in rats. *Cancer Res., 43*, 2477s-2484s.

Rogers, A.E. and Newberne, P.M. (1971). Diet and aflatoxin B1 toxicity in rats. *Toxicol. Appl. Pharmacol., 20*, 113-121.

Rose, A.L., Wen, G.Y., and Cammer, W. (1981). Hexachlorophene retinopathy in suckling rats. A light- and electron-microscopic study of short-term and long-term effect of hexachlorphene intoxication on the retina of young rats. *J. Neurol. Sci., 52*, 163-178.

Rosenkranz, H.S. and Leifer, Z. (1980). Determining the DNA-modifying activity of chemicals using DNA polymerase-deficient *Escherichia coli*. In *Chemical Mutagens, Principles and Methods for Their Detection*, Vol. 6, (F.J. de Serres and A. Hollander, eds.), pp. 109-147, Plenum Press, New York.

Rosenkranz, H.S. and Poirer, L.A. (1979). Evaluation of the mutagenicity and DNA-modifying activity of carcinogens and non-carcinogens in microbial systems. *J. Natl. Cancer Inst., 62*, 873-892.

Rossi, L., Ravera, M., Repetii, G. and Santi, L. (1977). Long-term administration of DDT or phenobarbital in Wistar rats. *Int. J. Cancer, 19*, 179-185.

Saccharin Hydrolysis Products (1982). Report from the Sherwin Williams Company Technical Department, Cincinnati, Ohio, May 26, 1982.

Saffiotti, U., Donovan, P. and Rice, J. (1979). Interactions of multiple carcinogens in the *Salmonella* mutagenesis assay (Ames). *AACR Abstracts*, March, p.191.

Sake, S., Reinhold, C.E., Wirth, P.J. and Thorgeirsson, S.S. (1978). Mechanism of *in vitro* mutagenic activation and covalent binding of N-hydroxy-2-acetylaminofluorene in isolated liver cell nuclei from rat and mouse. *Cancer Res., 38*, 2058-2067.

Salerno, R.A., Whitmire, C.E., Garcia, I.M. and Huebner, R.J. (1972). Chemical carcinogenesis in mice inhibited by interferon. *Nature, 239*, 31-32.

San, R.H.C. and Stich, H.S. (1982). Measurement of DNA repair synthesis in cultured human fibroblasts as a short-term bioassay for chemical carcinogens and carcinogenic mixtures. In *Cytogenetic Assays for Environmental Mutagens* (T.C. Hui, ed.), pp. 234-248, Allenheld, New Jersey.

Saxholm, H.J.K., Iverson, O.H., Reith, A. and Brogger, A. (1979). Carcinogenesis testing of saccharin. No transformation or increased sister chromatid exchange observed in two mammalian cell systems. *Eur. J. Cancer, 15*, 509-513.

Sbrana, I., Rusciano, D., Lascialfari, D., Lari, T. and Loprieno, N. (1980). Cytogenetic and genotoxic studies on rabbits, cattle, mice, rats and human cells accidentally or experimentally exposed to the dioxin TCDD. *Atti Assoc. Genet. Ital., 26*, 233-276.

Schand, D.G., Mitchell, J.R. and Oates, J.A. (1975). *Handbuch der Experimentellen Pharmakologie* (O. Eichler, A. Farah, H. Herken and A.D. Welch, eds.), pp. 272-314, Springer-Verlag, Berlin.

Schechter, B. and Feldman, M. (1979). Suppressor cells prevent host resistance to tumor growth. *Naturwissenschaften, 66*, 140-146.

Schevins, L.E., Mayersbach, H. and Pauly, J.E. (1974). An overview of chrono-pharmacology. *J. Eur. Toxicol., 7*, 203-227.

Schneider, R.P. (1975). Mechanism of inhibition of rat brain sodium, potassium-adenosine tri-phosphatase by 2,2-bis(p-chlorophenyl)-1,1,1-trichloroethane (DDT). *Biochem. Pharmacol., 24*, 939-946.

Schoenig, G.P. and Anderson, R.L. (1984). The effect of high dietary levels of sodium saccharin on selected physiological parameters in rats. *Food Chem. Toxicol.*, (Submitted for publication).

Schoenig, G.P., Goldenthal, E.I., Geil, R.G., Frith, C.H., Richter, W.R. and Carlborg, F.W. (1984). Evaluation of the dose-response and *in utero* exposure of saccharin in the rat. *Food Chem. Toxicol.*, (Submitted for publication).

Schrenk, H.H., Yant, W.P., Pearce, S.J., Patty, F.A. and Sayers, R.R. (1941). Absorption, distribution and elimination of benzene by body tissues and fluids of dogs exposed to benzene vapor. *J. Ind. Hyg. Toxicol.*, *23*, 20-34.

Schreck, R. (1979). *In vivo* induction of sister chromatid exchanges in liver and marrow cells by drugs requiring metabolic activation. *Mutat Res.*, *64*, 315-328.

Schreiber, H., Nettesheim, P., Lijinsky, W., Richter, C.B. and Walburg, H.E. (1972). Induction of lung cancer in germfree, specific-pathogen-free, and infected rats by N-nitrosoheptamethyleneimine. Enhancement by respiratory infection. *J. Natl. Cancer Inst.*, *49*, 1107-1114.

Schumann, A.M. and Watanabe, P.G. (1979). Species differences between rats and mice on the metabolism and hepatic macromolecular binding of tetrachloroethylene. *Toxicol. Appl. Pharmacol.*, *48*, A89.

Schumann, A.M., Quast, T.F. and Watanabe, P.G. (1980). The pharmacokinetics and macromolecular interactions of perchloroethylene in mice and rats as related to oncogenicity. *Toxicol. Appl. Pharmacol.*, *55*, 207-219.

Schupbach, M. and Hummler H. (1977). A comparative study on the mutagenicity of ethylenethiourea in bacterial and mammalian test systems. *Mutat. Res.*, *56*, 111-120.

Schwandt, P., Klinge, O. and Immich, H. (1978). Clofibrate and the liver. *Lancet*, *2*, 325.

Schwartz, A.G. and Moore, C.J. (1977). Inverse correlation between species life span and capacity of cultured fibroblasts to bind 7,12-dimethylbenz(a)-anthracene to DNA. *Exper. Cell Res.*, *109*, 448.

Schwartz, A.G. and Moore, C.J. (1979). Inverse correlation between species life span and capacity of cultured fibroblasts to metabolize polycyclic hydrocarbon carcinogens. *Fed. Proc.*, *38*, 1989-1992.

Schwartz, P.E., LiVolsi, V.A., Hildreth, N., MacLusky, N.J., Naftolin, F.N., and Eisenfeld, A.J. (1982). Estrogen receptors in ovarian epithelial carcinoma. *Obstet. Gynecol.*, *59*, 229-238.

Schwetz, B.A., Leong, B.K.J. and Gehring, P.J. (1975). The effect of maternally inhaled trichloroethylene, perchloroethylene, methyl chloroform, and methylene chloride on embryonal and fetal development in mice and rats. *Toxicol. Appl. Pharmacol.*, *32*, 84-96.

Schwetz, B.A., Norris, J.M., Sparchu, G.L., Rowe, V.K., Gehring, P.J., Emerson, J.L. and Gerbig, C.G. (1973). Toxicology of chlorinated dibenzo-p-dioxins. *Environ. Health Perspect.*, *5*, 87-99.

Seiler, J. (1973). A survey on the mutagenicity of various pesticides. *Experientia*, *29*, 622-623.

Seiler, J. (1977). Inhibition of testicular DNA synthesis by chemical mutagens and carcinogens. Preliminary results in the validation of a more short-term test. *Mutat. Res.*, *46*, 305-310.

Selgrade, M.K., Ahmed, A., Sell, K.W., Gershwin, M.E. and Steinberg, A.D. (1976). Effect of murine cytomegalovirus on the *in vitro* responses of T and B cells to mitogens. *J. Immunol., 116*, 1459-1465.

Shahin, J. and Fournier, F. (1978). Suppression of mutation induction and failure to detect mutagenic activity with athabascan tar sand fractions. *Mutat. Res., 58*, 29-34.

Shavit, Y., Lewis, J.W., Terman, G.W., Gale, R.P. and Liebeskind, J.C. (1984). Opioid peptides mediate the suppressive effect of stress on natural killer cell cytotoxicity. *Science, 223*, 188-190.

Sheiness, D. and Bishop, J.M. (1979). DNA from uninfected vertebrate cells contain nucleic acid sequences related to the putative transforming gene of avian myelocytomatosis virus. *J. Virol., 31*, 514-521.

Shih, C., Shilo, B. and Goldfarb, M.P. (1979). Passage of phenotypes of chemically transformed cells via transfection of DNA and chromatin. *Proc. Natl. Acad. Sci. U.S.A., 76*, 5714-5718.

Shih, C. and Weinberg, R.A. (1982). Isolation of a transforming sequence from a human bladder carcinoma cell line. *Cell, 29*, 161-169.

Shiffman, S.S., Lindley, M.G., Clark, T. and Makino, C. (1981). Molecular mechanism of sweet taste: relationship of hydrogen bonding to taste sensitivity for both young and elderly. *Neurobiol. Aging, 2*, 173-175.

Shinozuka, J., Katyal, S.L. and Lombardi, B. (1978). Azaserine carcinogenesis: organ susceptibility change in rats fed a diet devoid of choline. *Int. J. Cancer, 22*, 36-39.

Sieber, S.M. and Adamson, R.H. (1978). Long-term studies on the potential carcinogenicity of artificial sweeteners in non-human primates. In *Health and Sugar Substitutes*, Proceedings of the ERGOB Conference on Sugar Substitute, Geneva, Switzerland.

Simmon, V.F. (1979a). *In vitro* assays for recombinogenic activity of chemical carcinogens and related compounds with *Saccharomyces cerevisiae* D3. *J. Natl. Cancer Inst., 62*, 901-909.

Simmon, V.F. (1979b). *In vitro* mutagenicity assays of chemical carcinogens and compounds with *Salmonella typhimurium. J. Natl. Cancer Inst., 62*, 893-899.

Simon, D., Yen, S. and Cole, P. (1975). Coffee drinking and cancer of the lower urinary tract. *J. Natl. Cancer Inst., 54*, 587-591.

Singer, B. and Kroger, M. (1979). Participation of modified nucleotides in translation and transcription. *Prog. Nucl. Acid Res. Mol. Biol., 23*, 151-194.

Sirover, M.A. and Loeb, L.A. (1976). Metal-induced infidelity during DNA synthesis. *Proc. Natl. Acad. Sci. U.S.A., 73*, 2331-2335.

Sivak, A. (1978). Mechanism of tumor promotion and carcinogenesis. A summary from one point of view. In *Mechanisms of Tumor Promotion and Cocarcinogenesis* (T.J. Slaga, R.K. Boutwell and A. Sivak, eds.), Vol. 2, pp. 553-564, Raven Press, New York.

Sivak, A. (1979). Examination of the effects of calcium pantothenate, sodium ascorbate, sodium saccharin and L-tryptophan as promoters of 3-methylcholanthrene-induced neoplastic transformation in BALB/c-3T3 cells. Report to Calorie Control Council by Arthur D. Little, Inc.

Sivak, A. (1982). An evaluation of assay procedures for detection of tumor promoters. *Mutat. Res., 98*, 377-387.

Sivak, A. and Tu, A.S. (1980). Factors influencing neoplastic transformation by chemical carcinogens in BALB/c-3T3 cells. In *The Predictive Value of In Vitro Short-term Screening Tests in Carcinogenicity Evaluation* (G.M. Williams, R. Kroes, H. W. Waaijers and K.W. van de Poll, eds.), Elsevier/North Holland, Amsterdam.

Siskind, G.W. (1974). Selective immune suppression using antigens and antibodies as pharmacologic agents. *Fed. Proc., 33*, 1886-1888.

Sklar, L.S. and Anisman, H. (1979). Stress and coping factors influence tumor growth. *Science, 205*, 513-515.

Sklar, L.S. and Anisman, H. (1980). Social stress influences tumor growth. *Psychosom. Med., 42*, 347-365.

Sklar, L.S. and Anisman, H. (1981). Stress and cancer. *Psychol. Bull., 89*, 369-406.

Slaga, T.J., Boutwell, R.K. and Sivak, A. (eds.) (1978). *Mechanisms of Tumor Promotion and Cocarcinogenesis*. Vol. 2, Raven Press, New York.

Smalley, H.E. and Radlett, R.D. (1970). Comparative toxicity of the herbicide paraquat in laboratory and farm animals. *Toxicol. Appl. Pharmacol., 17*, 305.

Smith, E.M., Meyer, W.J., and Blalock, J.E. (1982). Virus-induced corticosterone in hypophysectomized mice: a possible lymphoid adrenal axis. *Science, 218*, 1311-1312.

Smith, J.E. (1977). Inherited glutathione deficiency, model No. 94. In *Handbook: Animal Models of Human Disease Fasc. 6* (T.C. Jones, D.B. Hackel and G. Migaki, eds.), Registry of Comparative Pathology, Armed Forces Institute of Pathology, Washington, D.C.

Smith, R.L. (1973). Species variation in biliary excretion. In *Excretory Function of Bile*, Chapman and Hall, London.

Smith, R.L. and Caldwell, J. (1976). Drug metabolism in non-human primates. In *Drug Metabolism from Microbes to Man* (D.V. Parke, and R.L. Smith, eds.), p. 331-356, Taylor and Francis, London.

Snyder, C.A., Goldstein, B.D., Sellakumar, A.R., Albert, R.L. and Laskin, S. (1978a). The toxicity of inhaled benzene. (Abstr.) *Toxicol. Appl. Pharmacol., 45*, 265.

Snyder, C.A., Goldstein, B.D., Sellakumar, A.R., Wolman, S.R., Bromberg, I., Erlichman, M.N. and Laskin, S. (1978b). Hematotoxicity of inhaled benzene to Sprague-Dawley rats and AKR mice at 300 ppm. *J. Toxicol. Environ. Health, 4*, 605-618.

Snyder, C.A., Goldstein, B.D., Sellakumar, A.R., Bromberg, I., Laskin, S. and Albert, R.E. (1980). The inhalation toxicology of benzene: incidence of hematopoietic neoplasms and hematotoxicity in AKR/J and C57BL/6J mice. *Toxicol. Appl. Pharmacol., 54*, 323-331.

Snyder, R., Longacre, S.L., Witmer, C.M., Kocsis, J.J., Andrews, L.S. and Lee, E.W. (1981). Biochemical toxicology of benzene. In *Reviews in Biochemical Toxicology*, Vol. 3, (E. Hodgson, J.R. Bend and R.M. Philpot, eds.), pp. 123-153, Elsevier/North Holland, New York.

Society of Toxicology (1981). Re-examination of the ED01 study overview. *Fund. Appl. Toxicol., 1*, 26-128.

Solleveld, H.A., Haseman, J.K. and McConnell, E.E. (1983). Lifespan or two-year studies for carcinogenicity testing? An easy choice when using the Fischer 344 rat as a test animal. American College of Veterinary Pathology, 34th Annual Meeting, San Antonio, Texas.

Spector, D.H., Varmus, J.E. and Bishop, J.M. (1978). Nucleotide sequences related to the transforming gene of avian sarcoma virus are present in DNA of uninfected vertebrates. *Proc. Natl. Acad. Sci. U.S.A., 75*, 4102-4106.

Squire, R.A. (1981a). Human risk assessment from animal data. In *The Pesticide Chemist and Modern Toxicology*, American Chemical Society Symposium Series 160 (S.K. Bandal, G.J. Marco, L. Golberg and M.L. Leng, eds.), pp. 494-501, American Chemical Society, Washington, D.C.

Squire, R.A. (1981b). Ranking carcinogens: a proposed regulatory approach. *Science, 214*, 877-880.

Sram, R.J. and Benes, V. (1974). Mutagenicity testing of ethylenethiourea. Report for joint FAO/WHO meeting of pesticide residues.

Staffa, J.A., and Mehlman, M.A. (eds.) (1979). *Innovations in Cancer Risk Assessment* (ED01 Study) pp. 1-246. Pathotox Publishers, Park Forest South, Illinois.

Stehelin, D., Varmus, J.E., and Bishop, J.M. (1976). DNA related to the transforming gene(s) of avian sarcoma viruses is present in normal avain DNA. *Nature* (London), *260*, 170-173.

Stenger, R.J., Porway, M., Johnson, E.A. and Datta R.K. (1975). Effects of chlordane pretreatment on the hepatotoxicity of carbon tetrachloride. *Exp. Mol. Pathol., 23*, 144-153.

Stewart, R.D., Hake, C.L., Forster H.V., Lebron, A.J., Peterson, J.E. and Wu, A. (1974). *Methylene Chloride: Development of a Biologic Standard for the Industrial Worker by Breath Analysis*, Report No. NIOSH-MCOW-ENVM-MC 74-9. National Institute of Occupational Safety and Health, Cincinnati, Ohio.

Stich, H.F. and Klesser, D. (1974). Use of DNA repair synthesis in detecting organotropic actions of chemical carcinogens. *Proc. Soc. Exp. Biol. Med., 145*, 1339-1342.

Stich, H.F., San, R.H.C., Lam, P.P.S., Koropatnick, D.J., Lo, L.W. and Laishes, B.A.(1976). DNA fragmentation and DNA repair as an *in vitro* and *in vivo* assay for chemical procarcinogens, carcinogens and carcinogenic nitrosation products. In *Screening Tests in Chemical Carcinogenesis* (R. Montesano, H. Bartsch and L. Tomatis, eds.), p. 617, International Agency for Research on Cancer, Lyon.

Stier, A., Clauss, R. Lücke, A. and Reitz, I. (1980). Redox cycle of stable mixed nitroxides formed from carcinogenic aromatic amines. *Xenobiotica, 10*, 661-673.

Stine, G.J. (1973). Effects of nitrilotriacetic acid on development of *Neurospora crassa*. *Am. Soc. Microbiol., 73,* Abstract 31.

Stine, G.F. and Hardigree, A.A. (1972). Effect of nitrilotriacetic acid on growth and mating in strains of *Escherichia coli* K-12. *Can. J. Microbiol. 18*, 1159-1162.

Stoltz, D.R., Stavsic, B., Klaassen, R., Bendall, R.D. and Craig, J. (1977). The mutagenicity of saccharin impurities. I. Detection of mutagenic activity. *J. Environ. Pathol. Toxicol., 1*, 139-146.

Stone, D., Lamson, E., Chang, Y.S. and Pickering, K.W. (1969). Cytogenetic effects of cyclamates on human cells *in vitro. Science, 164*, 568-569.

Stoner, G.D., Kniazeff, A.J., Shimkin, M.B. and Hoppenstand, R.D. (1974). Suppression of chemically-induced pulmonary tumors by treatment of strain A mice with murine sarcoma virus. *J. Natl. Cancer Inst., 53*, 493-498.

Stott, W.T., Reitz, R.H., Schumann, A.M. and Watanabe, A.G. (1981). Genetic and non-genetic events in neoplasia. *Food Cosmet. Toxicol., 19*, 567-576.

Stout, D., Hemminki, K. and Becker, F. (1980). Covalent binding of 2-acetylamino-fluorene, 2-aminofluorene, and N-hydroxy-2-acetylaminofluorene to rat liver nuclear DNA and protein *in vivo* and *in vitro. Cancer Res., 40*, 3579-3584.

Svoboda, D.J. and Azarnoff, D.L. (1979). Tumors in male rats fed ethyl chlorophenoxy-isobutyrate, a hypolipidemic drug. *Cancer Res., 39*, 3419-3428.

Swaisband, A.J., Pierce, D.M. and Franklin, R.A. (1977). The disposition of a novel pyrimidoindole, ciclazindol, in the rat and patas monkey. *Drug Metab. Dispos., 5*, 419.

Sweatman, T.W. and Renwick, A.G. (1980). The tissue distribution and pharmacokinetics of saccharin in the rat. *Toxicol. Appl. Pharmacol., 55*, 18-31.

Sweatman, T.W. and Renwick, A.G. (1979). Saccharin metabolism and tumorigenicity. *Science, 205*, 1019-1020.

Sweatman, T.W., Renwick, A.G. and Burgess, C.D. (1981). The pharmacokinetics of saccharin in man. *Xenobiotica, 11*, 531-540.

Swenberg, J.A., Cooper, H.K., Bucheler, J. and Kleihues, P. (1979). 1,2-Dimethylhy-drazine-induced methylation of DNA bases in various rat organs and the effect of pretreatment with disulfiram. *Cancer Res., 39*, 465-467.

Sylvester, P., Aylsworth, C., Van Vugt, D., and Meites, J. (1983). Effects of alterations in early hormone environment on development and hormone dependency of carcinogen induced mammary tumors in rats. *Cancer Res., 43*, 5342-5346.

Tabin, C.J., Bradley, S.M., Bargmann, I.C., Weinberg, R.A. Papageorge, A.G., Scolnick, E.M., Dhar, R., Lowy, D.R. and Chang, E. H. (1982). Mechanism of activation of a human oncogene. *Nature, 300*, 143-149.

Takeishi, K., Kaneda, S.O. and Seno, T. (1979). Mutagenic activation of 2-acetyl-aminofluorene by guinea-pig liver homogenates: essential involvement of cytochrome P-450 mixed-function oxidases. *Mutat. Res., 62*, 425-437.

Takeyama, H., Kawashima, K., Yamada, K. and Ito, Y. (1979) Induction of tumor resistance in mice by L1210 leukemia cells persistently infected with HVJ (Sendai virus). *Gann, 70*, 493-501.

Talmadge, J.E., Meyers, K.M., Prieur, D.J. and Starkey, J.R. *(1980).* Role of NK cells in tumor growth and metastasis in beige mice. *Nature, 284,622-624.*

Tannenbaum, A. (1944). The dependence of the genesis of induced skin tumors on the caloric intake during different stages of carcinogenesis. *Cancer Res., 4*, 673-677.

Tannenbaum, A. and Silverstone, H. (1949). The genesis and growth of tumors. IV. Effects of varying the proportion of protein (casein) in the diet. *Cancer Res., 9*, 162-169.

Tannenbaum, A. and Silverstone, H. (1957). Nutrition and genesis of tumors. In *Cancer* (R.W. Raven, ed.), Vol. 1, p. 306, Butterworth, London.

Tannenbaum, S.R. and Skipper, P.L. (1983). Biological aspects to the evaluation of risk: dosimetry of carcinogens in man. Presented at International Life Sciences Institute Symposium on Safety Assessment, The Interface between Science Law and Regulation. Arlington, Virginia.

Tanooka, H. (1977). Development and applications of *Bacillus subtilis* test systems for mutagens involving DNA-repair deficiency and suppressible auxotrophic mutations. *Mutat. Res., 42*, 19-32.

Tarone, R.E. (1982). Use of historical control information in testing for a trend in proportions. *Biometrics, 38*, 215-220.

Tarone, R.E., Chu, K.C. and Ward, J.M. (1981). Variability in the rates of some naturally occurring tumors in Fischer 344 rats and (C57BL/6N x C3H/HeN)F1-(B6C3F1) mice. *J. Natl. Cancer Inst., 66*, 1175-1181.

Task Force of Past Presidents (1982). Animal data in hazard evaluation: paths and pitfalls. Task Force of Past Presidents of the Society of Toxicology. *Fundam. Appl. Toxicol., 2*, 101-107.

Taylor, J.M., Weinberger, M.A. and Friedman, L. (1980). Chronic toxicity and carcinogenicity to the urinary bladder of sodium saccharin in the *in utero*-exposed rat. *Toxicol. Appl. Pharmacol., 54*, 57-75.

Telang, S. Tong, C. and Williams, G.M. (1982). Epigenetic membrane effects of a possible tumor promoting type on cultured liver cells by the non-genotoxic organochlorine pesticides chlordane and heptachlor. *Carcinogenesis, 3*, 1175-1178.

Teramoto, S. Moriyo, M., Kato, K., Tezuka, H., Nahamura, S., Shigu, A. and Shirasu, Y. (1977). Mutagenicity testing of ethylenethiourea. *Mutat. Res., 56*, 121-129.

Terracini, B., Testa, M.C., Cabral, J.R. and Day, N. (1973). The effects of long-term feeding of DDT to BALB/c mice. *Int. J. Cancer, 11*, 747-764.

Testa, B. and Jenner, P. (1976). Induction and inhibition of drug metabolizing enzyme systems. In *Drug Metabolism: Chemical and Biochemical Aspects*, (B. Testa and P. Jenner, eds.), p. 329, Marcel Dekker, New York.

Theiss, J.C., Shimkin, M.B., Stoner, G.D., Kniazeff, A.J., and Hoppenstand, R.D. (1980). Effect of lactate dehydrogenase virus on chemically-induced mouse lung tumorigenesis. *Cancer Res., 40*, 64-66.

Theiss, J.C., Stoner, G.D. and Kniazeff, A.J. (1978). Effect of reovirus infection on pulmonary tumor response to urethane in strain A mice. *J. Natl. Cancer Inst., 61*, 131-134.

Theiss, J.C., Stoner, G.D., Shimkin, M.B. and Weisburger, E.K. (1977). Test for carcinogenicity of organic contaminants of United States drinking waters by pulmonary tumor response in strain A mice. *Cancer Res., 37*, 2717-2710.

Thomas, C., Steinhardt, H.J., Kûchemann, K., Maas, D. and Riede, U.N. (1977). Soft tissue tumors in the rat. *Current Topics Pathol., 64*, 129-176.

Thompson, M.M. and Mayer, J., (1959). Hypoglycemic effects of saccharin in experimental animals. *Am. J. Clin. Nutr., 7*, 80-85.

Tisdel, M.O., Nees, P.O., Harris, D.L. and Derse, P.H. (1974). Long-term feeding of saccharin in rats. In *Symposium Sweeteners* (G.E. Inglett, ed.), pp. 145-158, Avi Publishing, Westport, Connecticut.

Tomatis, L. (1977a). Letters to the editor. Comment on methodology and interpretation of results. *J. Natl. Cancer Inst., 59*. 1341.

Tomatis, L. (1977b). The value of long-term testing for the implementation of primary prevention. In *Origins of Human Cancer* (H.H. Hiatt, J.D. Watson, and J.A. Winsten, eds.), Cold Spring Harbor Laboratory, New York.

Tomatis, L. (1979). The predictive value of rodent carcinogenicity tests in the evaluation of human risks. *Ann. Rev. Pharmacol. Toxicol., 19*, 511-530.

Tomatis, L., Agthe, C., Bartsch, J. Huff, J., Montesano, R., Sarracci, R., Walker, E. and Wilbourn, J. (1978). Evaluation of the carcinogenicity of chemicals: a review of the monograph program of the International Agency for Research on Cancer (1971 to 1977). *Cancer Res., 38*, 877-885.

Tomatis, L., Turusov, V., Day, N. and Charles, R.T. (1972). The effect of long-term exposure to DDT on CF-1 mice. *Int. J. Cancer, 10*, 489-506.

Tong, C., Fazio, M. and Williams, G.M. (1981). Rat hepatocyte-mediated mutagenesis of human cells by carcinogenic polycyclic aromatic hydrocarbons but not organochlorine pesticides. *Proc. Soc. Exp. Biol. Med., 167*, 572-575.

Toolan, H.W., Rhode, S.L. and Gierthy, J.F. (1982). Inhibition of 7,12-dimethylbenz(a)-anthracene-induced tumors in Syrian hamsters by prior infection with H-1 parvovirus. *Cancer Res., 42*, 2552-2555.

Toth, K., Somtai-Relle, S., Sugar, J. and Bence, J. (1979). Carcinogenicity testing of herbicide 2,4,5-trichlorophenoxyethanol containing dioxin and of pure dioxin in Swiss mice. *Nature, 278*, 548-549.

Trotter, J.R. (1980). Spontaneous cancer and its possible relationship to oxygen metabolism. *Proc. Natl. Acad. Sci. U.S.A., 77*, 1763-1767.

Trosko, J.E., Yotti, L.P., Dawson, B. and Chang, C.C. (1981). *In vitro* assay for tumor promoters. In *Evaluation of Short Term Tests for Carcinogens* (F.J. de Serres and J. Ashby, eds.), pp. 420-427, Elsevier/North Holland, New York.

Tucker, M.J. (1979). The effect of long-term food restriction of tumors in rodents. *Int. J. Cancer, 23*, 803-815.

Tunek, A., Platt, K.L., Przybylski, M. and Oesch, F. (1980). Multi-step metabolic activation of benzene: effect of superoxide dismutase on covalent binding to microsomal macromolecules and identification of glutathione conjugates using high pressure liquid chromatography and field desorption mass spectrometry. *Chem-Biol. Interact., 33*, 1-18.

Turusov, V.S., Day, N.E., Tomatis, L., Gatti, E. and Charles, R.T. (1973). Tumors in CF-1 mice exposed for six consecutive generations to DDT. *J. Natl. Cancer Inst., 51*, 983-997.

Uehleke, H., Werner, T., Greim, H. and Kramer, M. (1977). Metabolic activation of haloalkanes and *in vitro* tests for mutagenicity. *Xenobiotica, 7*, 393-400.

Ulland, B., Weisburger, J., Weisburger, E., Rice, J., Cypher, R. (1972). Thyroid cancer in rats from ethylenethiourea. *J. Natl. Cancer Inst., 49*, 483-484.

Umeda, M., Noda, K. and Ono, T. (1980). Inhibition of metabolic cooperation in Chinese hamster cells by various chemicals including tumor promoters. *Gann, 71*, 614.

U.S. EPA Workshop on Short-Term Bioassay for Estimating Carcinogenic Risk (1982). *J. Am. Coll. Toxicol., 1*, 185-186.

Upton, A.C., Clayson, D.B., Jansen, J.D., Rosenkranz, H. and Williams, G.M. (1984). Report of ICPEMC Task Group on the differentiation between genotoxic and non-genotoxic carcinogens. *Mutat. Res.,* in press.

Valencia, R. and Houtchens, K. (1981). Mutagenic activity of 10 coded compounds in the *Drosophila* sex-linked recessive lethal test. In *Evaluation of Short Term Tests for Carcinogens* (F.J. de Serres and J. Ashby, eds.), Elsevier/North Holland, New York.

van Abbé, N., Green, T., Jones, E., Richold, M. and Roe, F.J.C. (1982). Bacterial mutagenicity studies on chloroform *in vitro*. *Food Chem. Toxicol., 20*, 557-561.

Van Dijck, R. and Van de Voorde, H. (1976). Mutagenicity versus carcinogenicity of organochlorine insecticides. *Med. Fac. Landbouniv. Rijksuniv. Gent., 41(2)*, 1491-1498.

van Duuren, B.L., Goldschmidt, B.M., Loewengart, G., Smith, A.C., Melchionne, S.M., Seldman, I. and Roth, D. (1979). Carcinogenicity of halogenated olefinic and aliphatic hydrocarbons in mice. *J. Natl. Cancer Inst., 63*, 1433-1439.

Van Miller, J.P., Lalich, J.J. and Allen, R.A. (1977). Incidence of neoplasms in rats exposed to low levels of 2,3,7,8-tetrachlorodibenzo-p-dioxin. *Chemosphere, 6*, 537-544.

Vesselinovitch, S.D. (1983). Liver tumor induction. *Toxicol. Pathol., 10*, 110-120.

Visintainer, M.A., Volpicelli, J.R. and Seligman, M.E. (1982). Tumor rejection in rats after inescapable or escapable shock. *Science, 216*, 437–439.

Vogel, E., Blijleven, W.G.H., Klapwijk, P.M. and Zijlstra, J.A. (1980). Some current perspectives of the application of *Drosophila* in the evaluation of carcinogens. In *The Predictive Value of In Vitro Short-Term Screening Tests in Carcinogenicity Evaluation* (G.M. Williams, R. Kroes, H.W. Waaijers and K.W. van de Poll, eds.), pp. 125-147, Elsevier/North Holland, Amsterdam.

Vonderhaar, B.K. and Greco, A.E. (1982). Effect of thyroid status development on spontaneous mammary tumors in primiparous C_3H mice. *Cancer Res., 42*, 4553-4561.

Vos, J.G., Moore, J.A. and Zinkl, J.G. (1973). Effect of 2,3,7,8-tetrachlorodibenzo-p-dioxin on the immune system of laboratory animals. *Environ. Health Perspect.,* 5, 149-162.

Walker, A.I.T., Thorpe, E. and Stevenson, D.E. (1973). The toxicity of dieldrin (HEOD). I. Long-term oral toxicity studies in mice. *Food Cosmet. Toxicol., 11,* 415-432.

Walker, C.A. (1978). Species differences in microsomal monooxygenase activities and their relationship to biological half-lives. *Drug Metab. Rev., 7,* 295-323.

Wallace, M.E. and Knights, P. (1976). Pilot study of the mutagenicity of DDT in mice. *Environ. Pollut., 11,* 217-222.

Wallenberg, P. and Ullrich, V. (1977). Characterization of the drug monoxygenase in the mouse small intestine. In *Microsomes and Drug Oxidations* (V. Ullrich, A. Hildebrandt, I. Roots, R.W. Estabrook and A.H. Conney, eds.), p. 675, Pergamon Press, New York.

Wallenstein, M.C. (1981). Role of sympathetic system in morphine-induced mydriasis in rat. *Am. J. Physiol., 241,* 130-135.

Ward, J.M., Weisburger, J.H., Yamamoto, R.S., Benhamin, T., Brown, C.A. and S. Weisburger, E.K. (1975). Long-term effect of benzene in C57BL/6N mice. *Arch. Environ. Health, 30,* 22-25.

Warner, N.L., Woodruff, M.F. and Burton, R.C. (1977). Inhibition of growth of lymphoid tumors in syngeneic athymic (nude) mice. *Int. J. Cancer, 20,* 146-155.

Warren, J.R., Simmon, V.F. and Reddy, J.K. (1980). Properties of hypolipidemic peroxisome proliferators in the lympocyte (^{3}H) thymidine and *Salmonella* mutagenesis assays. *Cancer Res., 40,* 36-41.

Wassom, J.S., Huff, J.E. and Loprieno, N. (1977). A review of the genetic toxicology of chlorinated dibenzo-p-dioxins. *Mutat. Res., 47,* 141-160.

Weinstein, I.B., Morowitz, R.A., Mufson, P.B., Ivanovich, V. and Greenebaum, E. (1982). Results and speculations related to studies on mechanisms of tumor promotion. In *Carcinogenesis* (E. Hecker, N.E. Fusenig, W. Kunz, F. Marks and H.W. Thielmann, eds.), Vol. 7, pp. 519-616, Raven Press, New York.

Weisbroth, S.H. and Peress, N. (1977). Ophthalmic lesions and dacryoadenitis: a naturally occurring aspect of sialodacryoadenitis virus infection of the laboratory rat. *Lab. Anim. Sci., 27,* 466-473.

Weisburger, E.K. (1977). Carcinogenicity studies on halogenated hydrocarbons. *Environ. Health Perspect., 21,* 7-16.

Weisburger, E.K. and Weisburger, J.H. (1958). Chemistry carcinogenicity and metabolism of 2-fluorenamine and related compounds. *Adv. Cancer Res., 5,* 331-431.

Weisburger, J.H. (1964). Activation and detoxification of N-2-fluorenylacetamide in man. *Cancer Res., 24,* 475-479.

Weisburger, J.H. and Williams, G.M. (1978). Decision point approach for carcinogen testing. In *Structural Correlation of Carcinogenesis and Mutagenesis* (I.M. Asher and C. Zervos, eds.), pp. 45-52, The Office of Science, Food and Drug Administration, Rockville, Maryland.

Weisburger, J.H. and Williams, G.M. (1980). Chemical carcinogens. In *Toxicology: The Basic Science of Poisons*, 2nd Edition (J. Doull, C.D. Klaassen and M.O. Amdur, eds.), pp. 84-138, MacMillan Press, New York.

Weisburger, J.H. and Williams, G.M. (1982). Metabolism of chemical carcinogens. In *Cancer: A Comprehensive Treatise*, 2nd edition (F.F. Becker, ed.), pp. 241-333, Plenum Press, New York.

Weisburger, J.H. and Williams, G.M. (1984). Carcinogen bioassay in chemical carcinogens: *In vitro* and *in vivo* tests. In *Chemical Carcinogens* (C.E. Searle, ed.), American Chemical Society, Washington.

Weislow, O.S., Allen, P.T., Shepherd, R.E., Twardzik, D.R., Fowler, A.K. and Hellman, A. (1978). Protection against 7,12-dimethylbenz(a)anthracene-induced rat mammary carcinoma by infection with mouse xenotropic type C virus. *J. Natl. Cancer Inst., 61*, 123-129.

Weiss, J.M., Glazer, H.I., Phorecky, L.A., Brick, J., and Miller, N.E. (1975). Effects of chronic exposure to stressors on avoidance-escape behavior and on brain norepinephrine. *Psychosom. Med., 37*, 522-534.

Weisse, I., Stotzer, H., Kanppen, F. and Walland, A. (1971). The effect of clonidine on the pupil diameter and the retina in rats, assessed in relation to the intensity of light. *Arzneim.-Forsch., 6*, 821-825.

Weisse, I., Stotzer, H., Seitz, R. (1974). Age and light-dependent changes in the rat eye. *Virchows Arch. A., 362*, 145-156.

Welsch, C.W. and DeHoog, J.V. (1983). Retinoid feeding, hormone inhibition, and/or immune stimulation and the genesis of carcinogen-induced rat mammary carcinomas. *Cancer Res., 43*, 585-591.

Welsch, C.W. and Nagasawa, H. (1977). Prolactin and murine mammary tumorigenesis: a review. *Cancer Res., 37*, 951-963.

Welsh, R.M., Jr. (1978). Cytotoxic cells induced during lymphocytic choriomeningitis virus infection of mice. I. Characterization of natural killer cell induction. *J. Exp. Med., 148*, 163-181.

Welsh, R.M., Jr., Zinkernagel, R.M. and Hallenbeck, L.A. (1979). Cytotoxic cells induced during lymphocytic choriomeningitis virus infection of mice. II. Specificities of natural killer cells. *J. Immunol., 122*, 475-481.

Whitmire, C.E. (1973). Virus-chemical carcinogenesis: a possible viral immunologic influence on 3-methylcholanthrene sarcoma induction. *J. Natl. Cancer Inst., 51*, 473-478.

Whitmire, C.E. and Salerno, R.A. (1973). Influence of preinfection of C57BL/6 mice with Graffi leukemia virus on 3-methylcholanthrene-induced subcutaneous sarcoma. *Proc. Soc. Exp. Biol. Med., 14*, 674-679.

Wilkinson, C.F. (1976). Insecticide interactions. In *Insecticide Biochemistry and Physiology* (C.F. Wilkinson, ed.) p. 1605, Plenum Press, New York.

Williams, G.M. (1976). Carcinogen-induced DNA repair in primary rat liver cell cultures: a possible screen for chemical carcinogens. *Cancer Lett., 1*, 231-236.

Williams, G.M. (1977). Detection of chemical carcinogens by unscheduled DNA-synthesis in rat liver primary cell cultures. *Cancer Res., 37*, 1845-1851.

Williams, G.M. (1979a). Review of *in vitro* test system using DNA damage and repair for screening of chemical carcinogens. *J. Assoc. Off. Anal. Chem., 62*, 857-863.

Williams, G.M. (1979b). Liver cell culture systems for the study of hepatocarcinogenesis. In *Advances in Medical Oncology, Research and Education.Proceedings of the XIIth International Cancer Congress. Vol 1, Carcinogenesis.* (G.P. Margison, ed.), pp. 273-280, Pergamon Press, New York.

Williams, G.M. (1980a). The predictive value of DNA damage and repair assays for carcinogenicity. In *The Predictive Value of In Vitro Short-Term Screening Tests in Carcinogenicity Evaluation.* (G.M. Williams, R. Kroes, H.W. Waaijers and K.W. van de Poll, eds.), pp. 213-230, Elsevier/North Holland, Amsterdam.

Williams, G.M. (1980b). Classification of genotoxic and epigenetic hepatocarcinogens using liver culture assays. *Ann. N.Y. Acad. Sci., 349*, 273-282.

Williams, G.M., (1980c). The detection of chemical mutagens/carcinogens by DNA repair and mutagenesis in liver cultures. In *Chemical Mutagens, Principles and Methods for Their Detection,* Vol. 6, (F.J. de Serres and A. Hollander, eds.), pp. 61-79, Plenum Press, New York.

Williams, G.M. (1980d). Batteries of short-term tests for carcinogen screening. In *The Predictive Value of Short-term Screening Tests in Carcinogenicity Evaluation* (G.M. Williams, R. Kroes, H.W. Waaijers, and K.W. van de Poll, eds.), pp. 327-346, Elsevier/North Holland, Amsterdam.

Williams, G.M. (1981a). Epigenetic mechanism of action of carcinogenic organochlorine pesticides. In *The Pesticide Chemist and Modern Toxicology.* American Chemical Society Symposium Series 160 (S.K. Bandal, G.J. Marco, L. Golberg and M.L. Leng, eds.), pp. 45-56, American Chemical Society, Washington.

Williams, G.M. (1981b). Mammalian culture systems for the study of genetic effects of N-substituted aryl compounds. In *Carcinogenic and Mutagenic N-Substituted Aryl Compounds* (S.S. Thorgeirsson and E.K. Weisburger, eds.), pp. 237-242, National Cancer Institute Monograph, Washington.

Williams, G.M. (1981c). The detection of genotoxic chemicals in the hepatocyte primary culture/DNA repair test. In *Mutation Promotion and Transformation* (N. Inui, T. Kuroki, M.A. Yamada and E. Heidelberger, eds.), *Gann, 27*, 47-57.

Williams, G.M. (1981d). Liver carcinogenesis: the role for some chemicals of an epigenetic mechanism of liver-tumor promotion involving modification of the cell membrane. *Food Cosmet. Toxicol., 19*, 577-583.

Williams, G.M., Laspia, M.F. and Dunkel, V.C. (1982). Reliability of the hepatocyte primary culture/DNA repair test in testing of coded carcinogens and noncarcinogens. *Mutat. Res., 97*, 359-370.

Williams, G.M., Telang, S. and Tong, C. (1981). Inhibition of intercellular communication between liver cells by the liver tumor promoter 1,1,1-trichloro-2,2-bis(P-chlorophenyl)-ethane (DDT). *Cancer Lett., 11*, 339-344.

Williams, G.M. and Watanabe, K. (1978). Quantitative kinetics of development of N-2-fluorenylacetamide-induced, altered (hyperplastic) hepatocellular foci resistant to iron accumulation and of their reversion or persistence following removal of carcinogen. *J. Natl. Cancer Inst., 61*, 113-121.

Williams, G.M. and Weisburger, J.H. (1981). Systematic carcinogen testing through the decision point approach. *Ann. Rev. Pharmacol. Toxicol., 21*, 393-416.

Withey, J.R. (1982). Common pharmacokinetic mechanisms and considerations in species extrapolation. Presentation at a Workshop on Extrapolation to Man, December, 1982, Electric Power Research Institute, Palo Alto.

Witschi, H. and Lock, S. (1978). Butylated hydroxytoluene: a possible promoter of adenoma formation in mouse lung. In *Mechanisms of Tumor Promotion and Cocarcinogenesis* (T.J. Slaga, R.K. Boutwell and A. Sivak, eds.), Vol. 2, pp. 465-474, Raven Press, New York.

Witz, I.P., and Hanna, M.G., Jr. (1980). Contemporary topics in immunobiology. In *Site Expression of Tumor Immunity* Plenum Press, New York.

Wolff, S. (1981). The sister chromatid exchange test. In *Short-Term Tests for Chemical Carcinogens* (R.H.C. San and H.F. Stich, eds.), pp. 236-242, Springer-Verlag, New York.

Wolff, S. and Rodin, B. (1978). Saccharin-induced sister chromatid exchanges in Chinese hamster and human cells. *Science, 200*, 543-545.

Wolff, S. and Wiley, J. (eds.) (1982). *Sister Chromatid Exchange*, John Wiley and Sons, New York.

WHO (World Health Organization) (1967). *Procedures for Investigating Intentional and Unintentional Food Additives.* Technical Report Series, No. 348, p. 25, World Health Organization, Geneva.

WHO (World Health Organization) (1978). Principles and methods for evaluating toxicity of chemicals, Part 1. *Environmental Health Criteria* , Vol. 6, World Health Organization, Geneva.

Wright, A.S. (1980). The role of metabolism in chemical mutagenesis and chemical carcinogenesis. *Mutat. Res., 75*, 215-241.

Wurtman, R.J. and Moskowitz, M.A. (1977). The pineal organ (first of two parts). *New Engl. J. Med., 296*, 1329-1386.

Wynder, E.L. and Goldsmith, R. (1977). The epidemiology of bladder cancer: a second look. *Cancer, 40*, 1246-1268.

Wynder, E.L. and Stellman, S.D. (1980). Artificial sweetener use and bladder cancer: a case control study. *Science, 207*, 1214-1216.

Wyrobek, A., Gordon, L. and Watchmaker, G. (1981). Effect of 17 chemical agents including six carcinogen/noncarcinogen pairs of sperm shape abnormalities in mice. In *Evaluation of Short-term Tests for Carcinogens* (F.J. de Serres and J. Ashby, eds.), Elsevier/North Holland, New York.

Yager, J.D. and Yager, R. (1980). Oral contraceptive steroids as promoters of hepatocarcinogenesis in female Sprague-Dawley rats. *Cancer Res., 40*, 3680-3685.

Yamagiwa, K. and Ichikawa, K. (1915). Ueber die kustliche erzeugung oon papillom. *Verh. Jpn. Pathol. Ges., 5*, 148-152.

Yllner, S. (1961). Urinary metabolites of ^{14}C-tetrachloroethylene in mice. *Nature* (London), *191*, 820.

Yokoro, K., Nakano, M., Ito, A., Nagao, K., Kodama, Y. and Hamada, K. (1977). Role of prolactin in rat mammary carcinogenesis: detection of carcinogenicity of low-dose carcinogens and of persisting dormant cancer cells. *J. Natl. Cancer Inst.,* *58*, 1777-1783.

Yotti, L.P., Chang, C.C. and Trosko, J.E. (1979). Elimination of metabolic cooperation in Chinese hamster cells by a tumor promoter. *Science, 206*, 1089-1091.

Zetterberg, G., (1970). Personal communication reported by S.S. Epstein. *Int. J. Environ. Studies, 3*, 13-21 (1972).

Zubroff, J. and Sarma, D.S.R. (1976). A non-radioactive method for measuring DNA damage and its repair in nonprofilerating tissue. *Anal. Biochem., 70*, 387-396.

The Use of Short-Term Tests for Mutagenicity and Carcinogenicity in Chemical Hazard Evaluation

Editor in Chief
Dr. Harold C. Grice, Scientific Coordinator, International Life Sciences Institute, Nepean, Ontario, Canada

Associate Editor
Dr. Daniel Krewski, Environmental Health Directorate, Health Protection Branch, Health and Welfare Canada, Ottawa, Ontario, Canada

Contributors

B.E. Butterworth, Ph.D.
Chemical Industry Institute of
  Toxicology
Research Triangle Park,
North Carolina, U.S.A.

G. Douglas, Ph.D.
Health Protection Branch
Health and Welfare Canada
Ottawa, Ontario, Canada

V.C. Dunkel, Ph.D.
Food and Drug Administration
Washington, D.C., U.S.A.

H.C. Grice, D.V.M., M.Sc., V.S.
International Life Sciences Institute
Nepean, Ontario, Canada

R. Haynes, Ph.D.
York University
Toronto, Ontario, Canada

J.C. Jensen, Ph.D.
National Food Institute
Soborg, Denmark

D. Krewski, Ph.D.
Health Protection Branch
Health and Welfare Canada
Ottawa, Ontario, Canada

R. Kroes, D.V.M., Ph.D.
National Institute of Public Health
  and Environmental Hygiene
Bilthoven, Netherlands

J.P. Lewkowski, Ph.D.
The Coca-Cola Company
Atlanta, Georgia, U.S.A.

S. Molinary, Ph.D.
PepsiCo, Inc.
Valhalla, New York, U.S.A.

V. Ray, Ph.D.
Pfizer, Inc.
Groton, Connecticut, U.S.A.

J.J. Roberts, Ph.D., D.Sc.
Institute of Cancer Research
Royal Cancer Hospital
Sutton, Surrey, England

G.M. Williams, M.D.
Naylor Dana Institute for Disease
  Prevention
American Health Foundation
Valhalla, New York, U.S.A.

Contents

I. Introduction

DNA plays a central role in controlling cell function and reproduction. Both theoretical considerations and experimental evidence indicate that alterations in DNA structure can lead to a variety of deleterious effects including cancer and genetic disease. Because of the high level of concern regarding these diseases, as well as the mounting costs of health care, assays designed to provide information on agents with the potential for damaging DNA have attracted considerable attention among scientists, laymen and public health authorities alike.

Advances in the field of molecular biology that allow the study of chemical effects at the cellular and molecular level have provided much valuable information regarding the potential carcinogenic and mutagenic properties of chemical agents.

These assays are of substantially shorter duration than long-term carcinogenicity bioassays, and have accordingly been termed "short-term tests." The end points measured in these tests range from biochemical parameters such as the formation of DNA adducts, to induction of DNA repair in target cells in the whole animal, to mutagenesis in cultured cells and even to the production of lung adenomas in mice in abbreviated *in vivo* bioassays. While the focus here is on the more established assays previously included in published guidelines, the potential value of the other systems should not be overlooked.

It must be recognized that the orientation of most guidelines is on tests capable of assessing potential carcinogenicity. However, there is a growing awareness that mutagenicity *per se* represents a potential health hazard irrespective of its possible association with any particular disease state. Short-term tests are also valuable in identifying agents that have the potential to affect germ cells and thereby produce heritable mutations.

The acceptance of short-term tests in the process of hazard evaluation has been characterized both by enthusiasm and reluctance. The enthusiastic support comes from those who consider that the tests serve a useful purpose as indicators of mutagenic activity and predictors of carcinogenic potential, and that these tests provide the tools to better understand the mode of action of carcinogens. Those who have been reluctant to accept the tests are concerned about the lack of correlation that has been observed between certain results in specific short-term tests and those in long-term bioassays. Cell culture assays cannot be expected to reflect the species, strain, sex and organ specificities observed in carcinogenic assays. Human cells show different behaviors in many respects *in vitro* as compared with animal cells, e.g., high stability of human genetic materials like chromosome resistance to chemical transformation in human cells *in vitro*. The weight of evidence indicates, however, that short-term tests do have predictive value in assessing carcinogenic potential. There are few, if any, examples of compounds that are positive in a variety of genotoxicity assays covering different end points which have not been shown to be carcinogenic in rodent models (Butterworth, 1979; San and Stich, 1980; Williams, 1980).

Short-term tests are currently widely used in several countries in concert with bioassay data for assessing carcinogenicity. Such tests are also used in industry as a rapid and inexpensive means of identifying substances which are likely to be carcinogenic, with clear positive results being likely to preclude further development of a product. Although over 100 short-term tests have been described (Hollstein *et al.*, 1979; IARC, 1980; Purchase, 1982), there is a fair degree of consistency among tests recommended by different agencies.

The purpose of this report is to review current recommendations for specific tests, consider a number of critical issues in the interpretation of short-term test data, and evaluate the utility of a battery of tests. An historical perspective in the development of short-term tests is provided in Section II. Current guidelines offered by both individual scientists and various organizations are reviewed in detail in Section III, with a brief discussion of emerging tests presented in Section IV. Some general guidelines for the construction of a suitable battery of tests are provided in Section V. Possible approaches to the interpretation of conflicting results in different short-term test systems as well as differences between test results obtained in short-term tests are considered in Section VI. The document concludes with a brief summary of the utility and uses of short-term tests in the process of overall hazard evaluation.

II. Development of Test Strategies

All available short-term tests have been developed by researchers with specific scientific interests. A number of investigators have proposed schemes employing combinations of such tests for assessing the mutagenicity and potential carcinogenicity of chemicals. These schemes evolved from on-going research and generally were tailored to meet the specific concerns of the substance of interest including drugs, food additives and environmental chemicals. The accumulated body of information has contributed significantly to the development of useful, practical approaches to specific problems and has helped to ensure the orderly evolution of appropriate sets of tests for the various products of concern.

The tests proposed by various investigators are presented in summary form in Table I. Bridges (1973, 1976) proposed a three-tiered testing protocol consisting of submammalian tests, mammalian cells *in vitro* and whole mammalian tests. This protocol was intended for the detection of potential carcinogens and mutagens. The submammalian tests included mutagenesis in microorganisms and *Drosophila*, mutagenesis models in mammalian cells and cell transformation. Meiotic and mitotic chromosome damage and the micronucleus test were included in the second tier. Tier III included specific locus and carcinogenicity tests. In 1974, Stoltz *et al.* evaluated the status of short-term tests and suggested that three end points appeared to merit further scrutiny as possible bioassay methods for the rapid detection of carcinogens. These were mutagenesis, DNA repair synthesis and cell transformation. The schemes proposed by Flamm (1974) and Green (1977) differed from Bridges in favoring the dominant lethal test in lieu of a test for chromosomal damage.

Bora (1976) proposed a complex hierarchical scheme which included tests for mutation induction in bacteria, yeast and mammalian cells in culture, DNA damage and repair in human and other mammalian cells, *in vitro* chromosomal aberrations, *in vivo* chromosomal aberrations or micronuclei formation, dominant lethal, heritable translocation in mammalian germ cells, chromosomal aberrations in exposed human populations, gene mutation in mammals (specific locus test) and finally an epidemiological study of an exposed human population.

Dean (1976) proposed a testing scheme for industrial chemicals which consisted of three phases. Phase 1, the initial predictive screen contained assays for mutagenesis in bacteria and mitotic gene conversion in yeast both with and without metabolic activation provided by rat liver S-9 preparations, cytotoxicity in cultured cells and *in vitro* and *in vivo* chromosome damage. Phase 2 consists of four tests for providing additional information on mutagenic activity and carcinogenic potential. The tests are mutagenesis in bacteria and yeast with liver S-9 preparations from mice and other species, a dominant lethal assay in male mice, an assay for gene mutation in mammalian cells and when available an assay for transformation in cultured cells. Phase 3 contains a series of tests for carcinogenesis and mutagenesis including the following: an *in vivo* assay of gene mutation, dominant lethal assays in male and female mice, an *in vivo* chromosome study in Chinese hamsters or mice or both, long-term

Table I. Short-Term Tests Proposed by Various Investigators

Investigator	Mutation				DNA Repair Synthesis		Chromosomal Aberrations			Cell Transformation	Germ Cell Effects			Sister Chromatid Exchange	
	Prokaryotes	Eukaryotic Micro-organisms	*Drosophila*	Mammalian Cells	Mammalian Cells	Prokaryocytes or Fungi and Plant	*In Vivo*	Mammalian Cells *In Vitro*	Micronucleus Test	Hamster Embryo or BHK Cells or Mouse 10T½	Dominant Lethal	Heritable Translocation	Specific Locus	Eukaryotic Micro-organisms or Insects	Mammalian Cells *In Vitro or In Vivo*
Bridges (1973, 1976)	X		X	X		X		X	X	X					
Stoltz *et al.* (1974)	X				X					X					
Flamm (1974)	X[1]	X	X	X											
Bora (1976)	X[1]	X		X			X[2]	X			X				
Dean (1976)[5]	X	X	X	X			X	X	X	X	X	X	X		
Green (1977)	X	X		X							X	X	X		

Reference								
Weisburger and Williams (1978, 1981)	X	X	X	X		X	X[7]	X
Ray (1979)	X	X	X		X		X	
Sobels (1980)	X	X[8]	X[8]		X[9]		X	
Waters et al. (1980)	X	X	X		X		X	X
de la Iglesia et al. (1980)	X[3]		X		X[4]		X	X
Ashby (1983)	X	X[4]		X[6]	X	X		
Dean (1983)	X	X[6]		X	X			

[1] To include host mediated bacterial and eukaryotic mutagenesis
[2] To include chromosomal aberrations in exposed humans
[3] To include host mediation
[4] Complementary assay
[5] Also considers *in vivo* assay for gene mutation
[6] See text for alternate tests
[7] Recommended as a supplementary test
[8] Either mutation in mammalian cells or sex-linked recessive lethal in *Drosophila*
[9] Optional

carcinogenicity studies in one or two species, and pharmacokinetic and biochemical studies at the subcellular level. The selection of procedures in this last phase would depend on the nature and distribution of the compound and on an assessment of data obtained in Phase 1 and 2.

Weisburger and Williams (1978) proposed a battery of short-term tests for carcinogen detection as part of a step-wise decision point approach. This battery was subsequently modified to include bacterial mutagenesis, mammalian cell DNA repair synthesis, mammalian cell mutagenesis, and sister chromatid exchange (SCE). Cell transformation was suggested as an optional test (Williams and Weisburger, 1981). The rationale for this battery was to provide systems with different metabolic capability and complementary end points. The inclusion of SCE and transformation was intended to permit the detection of nongenotoxic as well as genotoxic carcinogens.

The battery provides differing metabolic parameters by including, in addition to tests employing exogenous liver enzyme metabolism, others that provide intact cell metabolism by primary rat, mouse and hamster hepatocytes (Williams, 1977). The specific tests selected for each end point were those generally available and thus with a substantial data base.

Ray (1979) proposed a battery employing point or gene mutation in prokaryotes and mammalian cells, *in vivo* and *in vitro* chromosomal anomalies and cell transformation. Sobels (1980) proposed a minimal battery consisting of at least three tests: 1) a test for point mutation in bacteria, 2) two tests for point mutations in eukaryotes, or 3) one test for point mutation in eukaryotes and one test for the detection of chromosome aberrations in mammalian cells *in vitro*. It was further suggested that two different metabolic activation systems should be employed. Waters *et al.* (1980) suggested a phased approach to the evaluation of environmental agents as mutagens and potential carcinogens. This involved the sequential application of bioassays which are organized into a three-level matrix emphasizing, first, detection then confirmation and, finally, hazard assessment. The emphasis in the Phase 1 test battery is on the detection of point mutations and primary DNA damage in microbial species and the detection of chromosomal alterations in mammalian cells (preferably involving *in vivo* exposure). The Phase 2 battery is designed to verify the results of Phase 1 tests by employing more relevant genetic and related bioassays for the corresponding end points in mammalian cells in culture, plants, insects and mammals. For the purpose of defining, provisionally, a negative result for mutagenicity and presumptive carcinogenicity, Waters *et al.* (1980) suggest the "core" battery of short-term tests is most important. This battery should include tests for point mutation in microorganisms and gene mutation in mammalian cells in culture; a test for chromosomal alterations (preferably an *in vitro* test); a test for primary damage to DNA using mammalian (preferably human) cells in culture; and a test for oncogenic transformation *in vitro*.

De la Iglesia *et al.* (1980) described a "chamber" testing system in which a flexible battery is applied to candidate new drugs. According to the authors, the purpose of short-term testing in the drug industry is basically to accelerate the decision-making process for the development of potential therapeutic agents. Toxicology studies are conducted simultaneously, and an assessment of the genetic and toxicologic profile is made. Point mutation, host mediation and DNA damage/repair appraisals meet the objectives of the first chamber: 1) to detect direct-acting carcinogens, 2) to identify metabolically-activated carcinogens, and 3) to isolate primary damaging agents. The second chamber includes cell transformation as well as other tests for the establishment of: 1) low-level acting or weak carcinogens, 2) the level of promotion needed for tumor induction, and 3) target organ specificity. The final choice of specific tests for use in each chamber is a function of their feasibility, validity, and sensitivity for particular drug classes.

As part of a decision tree approach to testing mutagens and potential carcinogens, Ashby (1983) proposed the use of short-term *in vitro* and *in vivo* assays. In this approach, once a reproducible, statistically significant positive response has been observed in an established *in vitro* assay, further bioassays *in vitro* are not recommended. Rather, chemicals shown to be genotoxic *in vitro* and, in exceptional circumstances, agents established as inactive should then be administered to rodents to assess their likely genotoxic activity *in vivo*. Specifically, the mouse bone marrow micronucleus assay was suggested to be among the simplest of *in vivo* assays to conduct, but others should be acceptable if sufficiently well validated. In the case where a negative response is observed in the primary *Salmonella* assay (5 strains plus or minus S-9, preferably using a pre-incubation protocol), this response should be confirmed in an established complementary eukaryotic assay. In most cases, a mammalian cell gene mutation or chromosome aberration assay would be selected for this purpose.

Dean (1983) outlined the United Kingdom Environmental Mutagen Society (UKEMS) guidelines for mutagenicity testing. Recommended tests in the UKEMS basic package included the following:

- a test designed to demonstrate the induction of point mutations (base-pair change and frameshift mutations) in established bacterial test systems, conducted with and without the use of appropriate metabolic activation systems;
- a test designed to demonstrate the production of chromosome damage

in appropriate mammalian cells grown *in vitro* with and without the use of appropriate metabolic activation systems;

- an assay for the detection of the induction of mutations in mammalian cells grown *in vitro*; or,
- tests designed to detect recessive lethals in *Drosophila melanogaster*;
- a test designed to demonstrate the induction of chromosomal damage in the intact animal using either the micronucleus test or, preferably, metaphase analysis of bone marrow or other proliferative cells; or,
- a test designed to detect the induction of germ-cell damage as demonstrated by the dominant lethal test in the rat or mouse.

III. Review of Organization Guidelines

The guidelines proposed by various organizations are presented in Table II. The table includes all short-term tests which are either recommended by some organization of authority, are in widespread use, or are particularly desirable in terms of their scientific relevance. In Table II the tests are categorized first by end point:

(i)   mutation
(ii)   chromosomal aberrations
(iii)   DNA damage and repair
(iv)   cell transformation (morphological)
(v)   germ cell effects (heritable; indicators)
(vi)   SCE.

Subcategories are by biological complexity:

(i)   prokaryotes
(ii)   lower eukaryotes
(iii)   insects
(iv)   mammalian cells (*in vitro*)
(v)   mammalian cells (*in vivo*).

Although Table II includes most of the commonly used tests, several short-term tests that have been proposed by various organizations have been omitted. For example, although there are numerous assays for the detection of mutagenic effects of chemicals in plants (Lucier and Hook, 1978), their relevance for man is generally not appreciated. Such assays may, however, be useful in specialized roles such as in monitoring for environmental pollution *in situ*. Other omissions include those tests involving biochemical rather than biological end points, such as those involving DNA degradation or alteration in enzyme function. Similarly, biological tests of limited utilization such as the sebaceous gland and hamster cheek pouch tests are also not considered.

In some instances, the agencies listed in the tables indicate a base set of tests with acceptable alternatives. Some agencies provide the rationale for their choice or make relevant comments concerning the tests. The guidelines may be summarized as follows.

Food Safety Council (FSC) (1978). The composition of a battery of testing procedures selected by FSC depends on the problem area being considered, i.e., whether it will be used for one of the following purposes: 1) to predict possible carcinogenic activity as part of a sequence of testing in product development, 2) to set priorities for selecting chemicals for long-term bioassays, or 3) to determine the hazard rating of industrial chemicals.

The following criteria may be applied in selecting a battery of testing procedures:

a) ability to cover all possible genetic lesions;
b) coverage of all likely metabolic products;
c) adequate reproducibility of test results;
d) appropriateness of design permitting quantitative evaluation;
e) predictive value for human risk.

A pragmatic approach must be taken to solve the problem of determining the mutagenic potential of a substance. For this purpose the following battery of tests is suggested:

> *for in vitro mutagenicity.* 1) point mutations in microbial and mammalian cell tests incorporating *in vitro* activating systems, 2) chromosomal changes *in vitro* in cultured mammalian cells, and 3) unscheduled DNA synthesis and/or DNA repair in mammalian cells;
> *for indirect in vivo mutagenicity.* 1) point mutations by a host-mediated assay using microbial or mammalian cells, 2) testing of body fluids using microbial indicator systems;
> *for in vivo mutagenicity.* 1) chromosomal changes *in vivo* by direct cytogenetic analysis of metaphase figure, 2) micronucleus test, 3) dominant lethal test;
> *for in vitro mutagenicity/carcinogenicity.* 1) cell transformation using appropriate *in vitro* cultured mammalian or human cell lines.

If further exploration is to be undertaken, the additional investigations might include: 1) fungal eukaryotic systems for forward mutation or mitotic recombination, 2) chromosomal aberrations using an *in vivo*

Table II. Short-Term Tests Proposed by Various Organizations

| | Mutation | | | | | | | | | | | | | | | | DNA Repair Synthesis | | | | | | | |
| | Prokaryotes | | | Eukaryotic Micro-organisms | | | | | Insects | Mammalian Cells (in Vitro) | | | | | | Mammalian Cells (in Vivo) | Mammalian Cells (in Vitro) | | | | | Mammalian Cells (in Vivo) | | |
	Choice Permitted	Salmonella	E. Coli	Choice Permitted	S. Cerevisiae	S. Pombe	N. Crassa	A. Nidulans	Drosophila	Choice Permitted	L5178Y	CHO	V79	Human Lymphoblasts	Human Fibroblasts	Human Lymphocytes	Choice Permitted	Primary Rat Hepatocytes	Human Hepatocytes	Rat Tracheal Epithelial Cells	Human Broncheal Epithelial Cells	Choice Permitted	Rat Hepatocytes	Rat Tracheal Epithelial Cells
FSC (1978)	R[f]	X		R[f]					R[f]	R							X							
OSHA (1980)	R	R		R					R	R	R						R	R						
IARC (1980,1982)		R							X[e]	X[e]	R							R						
NCI (1981)	X			X					X	X							X							
U.K. (1981)		R							X	X	R						X							
EPA (Pesticides) (1982)	X			X					X	X							X							
FDA (Threshold) (1982)	X								X[c]	X							X							
FDA (Food Additive)[a]	X			R					X[b]	X	R						X	R						
Netherlands (1982)	X	R			X				X	X	R						X	R						
NTP (1982)		R																R						
State of California (1982)	R			R					R	R						R						R		
Japan (1983)	X								X	R	S					R	R S							
NAS-NRC (1983)		X							X	X	R	R					R	R					R	
OECD (1983)	R								S	S							S					S		
EEC	X	X		S					S	S							S					S		

Table II *(continued)*

	Eukaryotic Micro-organisms — S. Cerevisiae (Aneuploidy) Choice Permitted	Insects — Drosophila	CA Mammalian Cells (in Vitro) Choice Permitted	CHO	Human Lymphocytes	Human Fibroblasts	Other Cells	CA Mammalian Cells (in Vivo) Choice Permitted	Rodent Bone Marrow	Rodent Lymphocytes	Human Lymphocytes	Micronucleus	Cell Transformation Mammalian Cells (in Vitro) Choice Permitted	Hamster Embryo	Human Fibroblast	BHK Cells	Mouse 10T½	Mouse 3T3
FSC (1978)				X					X				X	X				
OSHA (1980)													X					
IARC (1980, 1982)		R	R					R					R					
NCI (1981)			R															
U.K. (1981)			X					X[f]										
EPA (Pesticides) (1982)								X										
FDA (Threshold) (1982)				R														
FDA (Food Additive)[a]			X			R							R[d]					
Netherlands (1982)	X		R										X					
NTP (1982)			R										R					
State of California (1982)			X					R					R					
Japan (1983)			X									X	S					
NAS-NRC (1983)			R															
OECD (1983)												R						
EEC	S		X					X					S					

Table II (*continued*)

	Sister Chromatid Exchange													Germ Cell Effects (Heritable)				Germ Cell Effects (Indicators)					
	Eukaryotic Micro-organisms		Insects	Mammalian Cells (*in Vitro*)						Mammalian Cells (*in Vivo*)				Mammalian Cells (*in Vitro*)				Mammalian Cells (*in Vivo*)					
	Choice Permitted	*S. Cerevisiae* (Aneuploidy)	*Drosophila*	Choice Permitted	CHO	Human Lymphocytes	Human Fibroblasts	Other Cells		Rodent Bone Marrow	Rodent Lymphocytes	Human Lymphocytes		Choice Permitted	Specific Locus	Heritable Translocation		Choice Permitted	Sperm Morphology	UDS in Spermatocytes	Cytogenetics	Dominant Lethal
FSC (1978)														R				R				
OSHA (1980)				R														R				
IARC (1980, 1982)																						
NCI (1981)																						
U.K. (1981)																						X^f
EPA (Pesticides) (1982)																X						X

FDA (Threshold) (1982)			
FDA (Food Additive)[a]			
Netherlands (1982)			
NTP (1982)		R	
State of California (1982)	S		S
Japan (1983)			
NAS-NRC (1983)			S
OECD (1983)			
EEC		S	S

*Choice Permitted. Certain guidelines specify a test type rather than a specific assay. Some agencies recommend this to allow for flexibility. Results from any of a number of assays would appear to be acceptable.

X—Required test.

R—Recommended, suggested, or acceptable (see detailed comments in text).

S—Supplementary.

[a] Toxicological Principles for Safety Assessment of Direct Food Additives and Color Additives Used in Food—Proposed.

[b] Optional unless compound has anti-microbial activity.

[c] Substitute for either bacterial or mammalian cell assay depending upon situation.

[d] Optional.

[e] Either mutation in mammalian cells *or* sex-linked recessive lethal in *Drosophila*.

[f] Choice of one of these assays.

mammalian system, e.g., cytogenetic analysis of post-meiotic spermatocytes or oocytes; analysis for sperm head abnormalities; exposure of
pregnant animals followed by transplantation of embryo cells to a
syngeneic host.

International Agency for Research on Cancer (IARC) (1980). The
IARC uses the data from short-term tests in the evaluation of the
carcinogenicity of the chemical. In the evaluation, attention is given to
four categories as follows:

DNA damage. DNA binding, DNA breakage, DNA repair, induction
of prophage in bacteria, positive response in survival of repair
proficient or deficient cells;

mutagenicity. refers to induction of mutation in cultured cells or in
organisms, e.g., heritable alterations in phenotype, recombinations,
gene conversion and specific-locus mutation;

chromosomal anomalies. induction of chromosomal aberrations, including breaks, gaps, rearrangements, micronuclei, SCE, and aneuploidy;

others. cell transformation, dominant lethal, sperm abnormality, mitochondrial mutation.

Tables were constructed from the results of the above tests in a number
of biological systems (as shown).

prokaryotes	DNA Damage	Mutation	Chromosomal Abnormalities	Other
fungi/ green plants				
insects				
mammalian cells (in vitro)				
humans (in vivo)				

Tests were judged to be '+' or '−' in one or more assays. The overall
evidence summarized in the table for a particular compound was judged to
fall into one of three categories.

Sufficient. Evidence was considered sufficient when there were at least
three positive results in at least two of three test systems measuring
DNA damage, mutagenicity or chromosomal effects. When two of

the positive tests were for the same genetic effect, they had to be derived from systems of different biological complexity.

Limited. Evidence was considered limited when there were at least two positive results, either for different end points or in systems representing two levels of biological complexity.

Inadequate. Evidence was considered inadequate when there were generally negative, or only one positive, test results. Up to two positive test results were considered inadequate if they were accompanied by two or more negative test results.

In establishing these categories, the IARC Working Group gave greater weight to the three primary end points described above. Within the categories no specific systems are given any greater weight except that a positive in a mammalian cell system is required for designation of the compound as showing sufficient evidence of activity.

National Cancer Institute (NCI) (1981). The National Cancer Institute shares responsibility for selecting the most significant chemicals for carcinogenicity testing by the National Toxicology Program (NTP), and, therefore, directs its effort to selecting compounds whose carcinogenic potential could best be evaluated in long-term rodent bioassays. This chemical selection process is performed primarily by the NCI Chemical Selection Working Group (CSWG), which consists of senior NCI staff and representatives from a number of other governmental agencies. Historically, it has been difficult, based only on available production, use pattern, and limited animal and epidemiological data, to determine from the multitude of chemicals in use those of sufficient socioeconomic impact and scientific concern to warrant lengthy and expensive chronic tests. Accordingly, data from two mutagenicity tests, the *Salmonella*/mammalian microsome assay and the L5178Y TK+/-mouse lymphoma assay, are being used to assist the CSWG in the chemical selection process.

Environmental Protection Agency (EPA): Pesticides Registration (1982). This proposed rule specifies the kinds of data and information that must be submitted to EPA to support the registration/reregistration or experimental use of each pesticide product under the Federal Insecticide Fungicide and Rodenticide Act (FIFRA). As part of the toxicology data requirements, a battery of mutagenicity tests is required if any of the following conditions are met: 1) the product is to be used on food or feed; 2) the product is likely to result in significant human exposure; or 3) the active ingredient(s) or any of its (their) metabolites is structurally related to a mutagen or oncogen or belongs to any chemical class of compound containing mutagens or oncogens.

The battery of mutagenicity assays must include tests to assess the potential to induce gene mutations, structural chromosome aberrations or other genotoxic effects. The latter can include DNA damage and repair, numerical chromosomal aberrations and target organ/cell analysis (sperm morphology, DNA synthesis inhibition, DNA alkylation).

Currently recognized tests in each of these categories are listed with the National Technical Information Service (NTIS). Selection of tests within the battery shall be supported and take into account the limitations of the individual assay. In addition, because of rapid improvement in the field, registrants are encouraged to discuss with the Agency test battery selection, protocol design and results of preliminary testing.

Food and Drug Administration (FDA) (Threshold Assessment) (1982a). The Threshold Assessment Guideline is used by FDA as a means of deciding which substances administered to food-producing animals might have the potential to contaminate edible tissues with residues that pose a carcinogenic risk. The procedure uses a decision tree approach which examines the chemical structure of the compound, the toxicological data on the agent including the results of *in vitro* mutagenicity studies, the use of the agent in food-producing animals and the residue level of the parent compound and/or its metabolites in edible tissue. The guideline does not require the use of specific *in vitro* tests but does recommend that the battery should test the ability of the compound to induce mutation in two test systems that have been demonstrated to have a high correlation between detected mutagens and positive results in lifetime bioassays for carcinogenicity. The tests recommended are:

1) a bacterial point mutation assay with and without metabolic activation;
2) a mammalian cell mutation assay with and without metabolic activation;
3) an assay for unscheduled DNA synthesis in mammalian cells in culture.

An assay for sex-linked recessive lethal in *Drosophila* can be substituted for either the bacterial or mammalian cell mutagenesis assays depending upon the particular situation.

Food and Drug Administration (Toxicological Principles for the Safety Assessment of Direct Food Additives and Color Additives Used in Food) (1982b). A battery of short-term tests for determining carcinogenic potential is proposed for use in the safety assessment of direct food additives and color additives. Although the principles set forth in this document apply to both new substances and those already regulated, the major application is for safety testing of new additives. New substances would be assigned to one of three concern levels based on population exposure and an initial estimate of toxicity from knowledge of their molecular structures. The concern levels are indicative of low, intermediate and high concern for safety and relate directly to minimum testing requirements. For each concern level, short-term tests are a baseline requirement. For compounds of either low or intermediate concern, a positive response in the battery of short-term tests would lead to a requirement for a carcinogenicity bioassay in either one or two rodent species. For compounds of higher concern, the results from the battery would be used for determining the sequence in which the animal bioassays would be conducted. In addition, the results from the *in vitro* battery could also aid in the evaluation of equivocal results from a carcinogenicity bioassay.

The *in vitro* tests identified for use in the battery include:

1) a bacterial mutagenesis test (the Ames test is suggested);
2) a mammalian cell mutagenesis test (the L5178Y mouse lymphoma assay is suggested); and
3) a test for unscheduled DNA synthesis (the primary rat hepatocyte assay is suggested).

Tests for *in vitro* transformation and sex-linked recessive lethal in *Drosophila* would be optional testing requirements.

Occupational Safety and Health Administration (OSHA) (1980). The OSHA Cancer Policy establishes the criteria and procedures under which individual substances, groups of substances or mixtures of substances, which may be found in the workplace will be regulated as potential occupational carcinogens. Such potential occupational carcinogens will be identified and classified on the basis of human epidemiological studies and/or experimental carcinogenesis bioassays. Positive results in short-term tests will be used as concordant evidence. The latter is defined as positive results in assays for two or more of the following types of effects:

1) the induction of DNA damage and/or repair;
2) mutagenesis in bacteria, yeast, *Neurospora* or *Drosophila melanogaster*;
3) mutagenesis in mammalian somatic cells;
4) mutagenesis in mammalian germinal cells, or
5) neoplastic transformation of mammalian cells in culture.

Netherlands (Health Council of the Netherlands) (1982). The following tests are recommended for mutagenicity and potential carcinogenicity. genicity.

Mutagenicity. A minimum package of three tests is recommended:

1) a test for gene or point mutation in prokaryotes;
2) one test in eukaryotic systems;
3) a choice between a test for the detection of point mutation or a test for the detection of chromosome abnormalities *in vitro*.

All *in vitro* tests should be conducted with and without metabolic activation. If these three tests are negative, the compound is assumed to be a mammalian nonmutagen. If positive results are obtained, further testing aimed at quantifying the possible mutagenic risk is required.

Carcinogenicity. For assessment of potential carcinogenicity, a DNA repair test and a cell transformation test are advised in addition to the minimum package for mutagenicity.

National Toxicology Program (NTP) (1982). The data obtained from short-term tests are considered important to the NTP from two aspects. The first is to provide information which can be used by the experimental design groups, and the second is for establishing the priority of chemicals to be entered into long-term carcinogenicity bioassays. The tests selected fall into five broad classes and include:

1) gene mutation in *Salmonella typhimurium*;
2) gene mutation in L5178Y mouse lymphoma cells (thymidine kinase);
3) *in vitro* cytogenetic damage and SCE in Chinese hamster ovary cells;
4) cell transformation in BALB/c 3T3 cells;
5) unscheduled DNA synthesis in primary rat hepatocytes.

This group of tests was chosen because the basic categories of genotoxic effects can be detected, the tests are readily available and the accepted protocols have been subjected to some form of evaluation or validation. The intention in the use of results from this group of assays is to obtain a reasonable profile of the genetic toxicity of a chemical.

State of California (1982). In addition to the federal requirements, one state, California, has suggested that short-term tests can be used to augment evidence for carcinogenicity from animal cancer bioassays that, for some reason, are not by themselves definitive. Short-term tests can also indicate the potential carcinogenic hazards of chemicals not yet tested in animals.

A battery of tests may be used including those which may assay the ability of the substance to cause:

1) gene mutation - bacteria, eukaryotic microorganisms, mammalian cells in culture or cells in intact animals (insects, mammals);
2) chromosomal aberrations, SCE, or formation of micronuclei in higher eukaryotes, including mammals;
3) induction of DNA repair in either *in vivo* or *in vitro* test systems; or
4) neoplastic transformation of cultured mammalian cells.

Japan (1983). The Japanese draft guidelines are intended to test for mutagens and potential carcinogens. The regulatory system in Japan follows the Organization of Economic Cooperation Development (OECD) guidelines in principle. For registration of new drugs, the Ames test and *in vitro* chromosomal aberration assay are required. If positive results are obtained in either or both of these tests, an *in vivo* test with mammals, such as the micronucleus test in mice, should be performed for confirmation. These tests are required at present in order to arrive at an assessment of mutagenicity. Other tests are employed as indicator tests shown in the tables. Screening tests for carcinogenicity employ the same tests. Presently in Japan, the Ames test is required for all kinds of chemicals. A guideline similar to that for drugs is being prepared for industrial chemicals, pesticides, food additives and other chemicals (Ishidate, 1983).

National Academy of Sciences—National Research Council (NAS-NRC) Committee on Chemical Environmental Mutagens (1983). This Committee addressed the topic of identifying and estimating the genetic impact of chemical mutagens. In approaching this problem, the committee defined its task as providing answers to two questions. (1) How can data from diverse test systems best be used to identify possible chemical mutagens and to assess their potential damage to human germ cells? (2) How can information on mutational damage produced by chemicals be used to estimate their possible impact on human welfare in future generations?

In answer to the first question, the committee suggested a two-tier system of short-term mutagenicity tests that could be applied widely to identify substances that may represent a mutagenic hazard. Tier I is composed of three tests:

1) *Salmonella*/microsome gene mutation,
2) mammalian cell gene mutation (HGPRT or TK locus), and
3) mammalian cell chromosome breakage.

All three tests should be conducted with and without metabolic activation. If all three tests are negative, the chemical is classified as a presumed mammalian nonmutagen. If two or all three of the tests are clearly positive, the chemical is classified as a presumed mammalian mutagen.

If both mammalian *in vitro* gene mutation tests (HGPRT⁻ and TK⁻) are done, and the result of either is positive, the committee recommended that the outcome in this test system be regarded as positive. Since the combination of positive results in one test and negative results in two tests is ambiguous, the system moves to Tier II. Tier II is composed of the *Drosophila* sex-linked recessive lethal test. If this test is positive, the substance is considered to be a presumed mammalian mutagen.

To answer the second question, the committee included tests for inherited point mutations and translocations *in vivo* in the mouse. From mouse data, perhaps combined with information from other tests, the effects in the first half-dozen human generations can be estimated, although with great uncertainty.

European Economic Community (EEC). The EEC guidelines are intended to test for mutagens and potential carcinogens. All new chemicals to be marketed in more than one metric ton per year are regulated by the sixth amendment to the 1967 directive.[1] For example, a new dye to be used in some industrial process would require testing before it could be legally placed on the market.

Substances which will be marketed in less than 10 metric tons per year (but more than one metric ton) are to be tested according to the base set of test requirements of the sixth amendment to the 1967 directive. The base set test requirements for short-term mutagenicity tests are:

1) one bacterial mutation test (*Salmonella typhimurium* or *Escherichia coli*);
2) one assay for chromosomal aberration in mammalian cells in culture; or one assay for chromosomal aberration in rodent bone marrow; or micronucleus test in rodent bone marrow.

If a substance is to be marketed in an amount of more than 10 metric tons per year, the authorities may require supplementary studies. A formal strategy for testing above the base level has not yet been developed, but the issue will be discussed at forthcoming meetings in the EEC. At present, the following tests have been described in test guidelines which will be published in the near future:

---

[1] Sixth amendment to the directive 67/548/18 September, 1979, EEC on the approximation of the laws, regulations and administrative provisions relating to the classification, packaging and labelling of dangerous substances.

- dominant lethal test,
- mouse heritable translocation test,
- mouse spot test,
- mouse specific locus test,
- bone marrow cytogenetics in rodents,
- mammalian germ cell cytogenetics and SCE in mammalian cells,
- sex-linked recessive lethal in *Drosophila melanogaster,*
- bacterial mutagenicity tests with *Salmonella typhimurium* and *Escherichia coli*,
- gene mutations,
- mitotic recombination and mitotic aneuploidy in *Saccharomyces cerevisiae*,
- gene mutation in *Schizosaccharomyces pombe*, and
- gene mutation and somatic segregation in *Aspergillus nidulans.*

Chemicals which are used as pesticides, food additives, feed additives or medicaments are, in addition, considered under other special regulations. For each of these four groups of chemicals, existing expert committees in the EEC review data and make recommendations regarding specific compounds under evaluation. No specific short-term test battery has been published from either of these committees, but short-term tests are, in general, required. Regarding food additives, the EEC expert group has published a report, part of which summarizes some general recommendations on the use of short-term tests in safety evaluation of food additives (EEC, 1980).

These test guidelines have been established with a view to avoiding major discrepancies between the EEC and the OECD guidelines.

Organization for Economic Cooperation Development (OECD) (1983). No specific battery of tests have been recommended as yet. However, only tests agreed upon by member countries as having utility are selected for the establishment of guidelines. In this context, guidelines refer to test protocols and not to a procedure for test deployment. The guidelines are intended to facilitate international trade to the extent that tests performed in one country would be considered valid in any other OECD country. Guidelines have been adopted for the following tests:

1) *Salmonella* mammalian microsome reverse mutation assay,
2) *Escherichia coli* reverse mutation,
3) *in vitro* chromosomal aberrations in mammalian cells,
4) *in vivo* micronucleus assay.

Guidelines have been written but not adopted for the following tests:

1) point mutation in cultured mammalian cells,

2) *in vivo* bone marrow chromosomal aberration in rodents,
3) dominant lethal assay in rodents,
4) sex-linked recessive lethal assay in *Drosophila*.

These tests have received various levels of approval by the OECD.

United Kingdom (U.K.)—Department of Health and Social Security—Guidelines for the Testing of Chemicals for Mutagenicity.Report of Committee on Mutagenicity of Chemicals in Food,Consumer Products and the Environment. (1981). Based on a number of considerations, this committee felt it was logical that before any assessment of a chemical can be made in terms of mutagenic hazard, it is essential to establish whether or not it can interact at the gene level in prokaryotes or eukaryotes (i.e., produce point mutations) and whether or not it can produce chromosomal damage in mammalian cells. For these purposes the committee developed a minimal or basic package of four screening procedures for mutagenic properties of chemicals.

1) A test designed to demonstrate the induction of point mutations (base-pair and frameshift mutations) in established bacterial test systems such as *Salmonella typhimurium, Escherichia coli* or *Bacillus subtilis*. The tests should be conducted with and without the use of appropriate metabolic activation systems.
2) A test designed to demonstrate the production of chromosome damage in appropriate mammalian cells grown *in vitro* with and without use of appropriate metabolic activation systems.
3) The induction of mutations in mammalian cells grown *in vitro*, or tests designed to induce recessive lethals in *Drosophila melanogaster*.
4) A test designed to demonstrate the induction of chromosomal damage in the intact animal using either the micronucleus test or, preferably, the metaphase analysis of bone marrow or other proliferative cells; or the induction of germ cell damage as demonstrated by the dominant lethal test in the rat or mouse.

It was the opinion of the committee that this recommended basic package screening procedure should detect, if fully and properly exploited, the great majority of potential mutagens among the chemicals entering the human environment. Any further improvement at the screening level would entail an expenditure of effort out of proportion to the value of the additional information that might be gained. The minimal package would be followed by supplementary tests that would be dictated by the kinds of results obtained, the kind of human exposure expected and factors such as the pharmacodynamics of the chemical involved.

Nordic Countries. Other countries which are members of OECD such as Norway and Sweden, have not yet come forward with specific test requirements or test guidelines concerning mutagenicity testing of chemicals, but, in general, these countries are in agreement with the OECD requirements.

The International Commission for Protection Against Mutagens and Carcinogens (ICPEMC). ICPEMC is an assembly of scientists whose objectives are to identify and promote scientific principles and to make recommendations that may serve as a basis for guidelines and regulations aimed at preventing or summarizing deleterious effects in man due to the interaction of chemicals with genetic material. Committee I of ICPEMC was specifically concerned with the validation, application and comparison of short-term screening systems for the identification and characterization of chemical mutagens. The committee selected 15 bioassays for evaluation as predictors of categories of genetic activity for a number of chemicals. These categories include nongenotoxic, genotoxic, mammalian germ cell mutagens and mammalian germ cell nonmutagens.

IV. Future Developments

The review of existing guidelines for the use of short-term tests shows that a variety of procedures are currently being used to evaluate chemicals for carcinogenic/mutagenic potential. However, the field is evolving and some existing tests are being modified and others are undergoing development.

Tests for chromosomal rearrangements, transposon movement and aneuploidy. There is increasing evidence that an important step in the development of some tumors is the unwanted expression of certain, otherwise normal, genes known as oncogenes. Such altered patterns of gene expression may be associated with specific chromosomal rearrangements or transposition events that change the genomic relationship between oncogenes and the regulatory sequences controlling them. Visible chromosome rearrangements induced by various chemicals have been studied for a long time in mutation research. Only a small, and probably specific, subset of these events would be expected to be involved in carcinogenesis since many induced chromosome aberrations are lethal. However, an important class of non-lethal rearrangements can be detected as mitotic recombination events in lower eukaryotes such as yeast, *Neurospora* and *Aspergillis*. It is for this reason that short-term tests based on these phenomena are continuing to be developed. Indeed, it is possible, when a sufficient data base is developed, that the ability of chemicals to induce mitotic recombination will correlate as well with carcinogenicity as induction of base-pair substitution mutations. In the past it has not been possible, apart from the observation of quadriradial chromosome configurations, to detect mitotic recombination in mammalian cells. The development of suitably marked cell lines for this purpose is a matter of some urgency.

A special category of chromosomal rearrangement is associated with the movement, or transposition, of mobile genetic elements known as transposons. A substantial fraction of spontaneous mutagenesis in organisms as diverse as bacteria, yeast and *Drosophila* has been attributed to transposon movement. Such elements can also alter patterns of gene expression and so may be involved in carcinogenesis. Unfortunately, there are few selective assay systems in which induced frequencies of transposon movement can be measured. (Where this is possible, it would appear that such frequencies are not much affected by "standard" mutagens.) However, in yeast, for example, the alcohol dehydrogenase system can be adapted for this purpose, and further work in this area should be monitored closely for possible application in genetic toxicology.

Aneuploidy, resulting from chromatid non-disjunction, is an important cause of genetic disease, and in somatic cells the resulting hemizygosis of recessive alleles might contribute to carcinogenesis. Indeed, it has been suggested that induced hemizygosis (or recessive homozygosis) could be an important step in tumor promotion. Because aneuploidy can be induced by attack on spindle protein, it is possible that certain nongenotoxic carcinogens act in this way. Certain otherwise nonmutagenic tumor promoters have been shown to be efficient inducers of aneuploidy in yeast (Parry *et al.*, 1981). Improved tests for aneuploidy are being developed in yeast (Dixon, 1983).

Measurement of DNA damage and repair. Carcinogens that form electrophilic reactants react with DNA and can be detected by *in vivo* covalent binding studies or measurement of DNA damage or repair (IARC, 1980; Lutz, 1979; Williams, 1983). The measurement of these end points in whole animals provides a means of assessing organ-specific toxicity and permits evaluation of factors such as compound uptake, distribution, metabolic activation, detoxification, DNA repair and excretion (Bridges *et al.* 1982). For example, the determination of chemically-induced DNA damage or DNA repair as measured by unscheduled DNA syntheses (UDS) are valuable tools that permit assessment of organ-specific genotoxic activity.

DNA damage. A variety of methods can be used to measure DNA damage induced by various agents (IARC, 1980). These include the detection of covalent binding or adducts in DNA using either radioactively labelled compounds (Lutz, 1979) or other techniques such as radio-immunoassay (Adamkiewicz *et al.*, 1982), fluorometric methods (Swenberg and Bedell, 1982) and post labelling methods (Gupta *et al.*, 1983). High pressure liquid chromatography/mass spectrometry techniques may prove sensitive for adduct detection (Farmer *et al.*, 1980). Adducts may also be detected and their loss monitored by the presence of sites in DNA sensitive to enzymes (or combinations of enzymes) that incise DNA at the site of damage and thus reduce its molecular weight.

Damage to DNA can lead to the formation of breaks in DNA directly or as repair intermediates, or to the formation of alkali labile sites in DNA. These changes to DNA can, therefore, be detected by changes in the size of single-stranded DNA, as measured either by alkaline sucrose gradient sedimentation or by alkaline elution (Bermudez *et al.*, 1983; Petzold and Swenberg, 1978).

An initial effect of many carcinogens is an inhibition of semiconservative DNA replication. Painter (1977) proposed an *in vitro* test for carcinogens based on this phenomenon. The test is simple and rapid but has not yet been extensively validated by comparison of related carcinogens and noncarcinogens.

As a consequence of the selective inhibition of DNA replication in which there is little or no effect on RNA or protein synthesis, cells treated with genotoxic agents often exhibit the phenomenon of unbalanced growth or giant cell formation. This phenomenon was considered by Grant and Grasso (1978) to be a possible screen for genotoxic agents.

The above effects on DNA replication can be further modified by posttreatment incubation of cells in the presence of a nontoxic dose of caffeine, a procedure that results in a dramatic increase in toxic and clastogenic damage to some cells (Roberts, 1976). Likewise, incubation of exposed cells with an inhibitor of DNA repair will potentiate the damage produced and reveal genotoxic effects in cells. However, neither of these effects has been validated as potential screening systems.

DNA repair. DNA repair is a natural response of the genetic material to chemical insult and occurs in most cells, is readily detected, does not require proliferating cells and can be measured in various cell types in culture or the whole animal. Larsen *et al.* (1982) considered the use of DNA repair in various *in vitro* and *in vivo* biological systems. One *in vivo* system (Mirsalis *et al.*, 1982b) detects UDS in primary rat hepatocyte cultures obtained from treated animals. This assay is valuable for some genotoxic nitro-aromatic carcinogens which require metabolism by gut flora for activation and are thus inactive in *in vitro* cell culture assays (Doolittle *et al.*, 1983b; Mirsalis and Butterworth, 1982; Mirsalis *et al.*, 1982a). Another advantage of the *in vivo–in vitro* approach is that it also detects cells in S-phase and can help distinguish between true genotoxic carcinogens and those that are only cytotoxic and induce cell turnover (Mirsalis *et al.*, 1982b). Germ cell DNA repair assays are available in the mouse (Sega, 1982) and rat (Working and Butterworth, 1982).

DNA repair also provides the means to begin bridging the gap between rodent models and the response in human beings. For example, DNA repair can be assessed in freshly isolated primary cultures of human hepatocytes (Butterworth *et al.*, 1983) and bronchial epithelium (Doolittle *et al.*, 1983a). These results can be contrasted to the response in rat hepatocytes (Williams, 1977) or hepatocytes from other species (McQueen *et al.*, 1983) and rat trachea (Doolittle and Butterworth, 1983).

Cell transformation. A number of cell transformation systems have been developed over the past decade (Heidelberger *et al.*, 1983; Meyer, 1983; Mishra *et al.*, 1980). Such systems permit study of the ability of carcinogens to convert nontumorigenic cells to a tumorigenic state or normal diploid cells to a pre-neoplastic state. The cellular mechanisms which underlie the process of transformation in these systems is not understood, but it is generally assumed that these systems are sensitive to the ability of chemicals to create cellular alterations which are causally related to malignancy. Such systems may possess sensitivity to carcinogens which act by mechanisms which will fail to elicit a response in other assays for genotoxicity.

The majority of the cell transformation systems used today utilize fibroblast cultures of embryonic origin. Such systems may use either permanent cell lines (BALB/c 3T3, BHK 21, C3H/10T$\frac{1}{2}$) or primary cultures of rodent embryo cells (Syrian hamster, rat or mouse). A system employing Syrian hamster fetal lungs is under development (Emura *et al.*, 1982; Grimmer *et al.*, 1983). Systems which utilize rat tracheal epithelial cells (Pai *et al.*, 1982) and human fibroblasts (Silinskas *et al.*, 1981) are realizing increased use, but are still in early stages of development. Also of interest is the development of assays for transformation in epithelial cells (Borek, 1983; Shimada *et al.*, 1983). Recent studies have suggested the mechanism of transformation may vary from system to system (Heidel-berger et al., 1983; Newbold et al., 1983), although it is not yet known which system(s) provide(s) information that is most relevant to the etiology of human cancer. The process of transformation within single systems can also be observed to proceed through stages analogous to initiation and promotion on mouse skin (Frazelle et al., 1983; Popescu et al., 1980; Sivak and Tu, 1980b). The use of multiple systems and/or different permutations of a single system may thus permit analysis of the ability of chemicals to accomplish different genetic and epigenetic aspects of the multi-step process of carcinogenesis.

Promotion. Although knowledge about mechanisms of carcinogenesis is still limited, it has become increasingly evident that cancer induction is a multi-step process. Since the early studies of Berenblum (1974) on two-stage induction of skin tumors (initiation/promotion), this process has become extended experimentally to other organs or tissues including liver, colon and urinary bladder. Essentially, certain requirements should be met in order to conclude that this is the functional process. These include:

- the initiation step and the promotion step should not overlap in time;
- neither one should be carcinogenic to any marked degree;
- augmentation should occur when the two agents are administered in one particular sequence but not in reverse order;
- extending the time between initiation and the promoting action should not lead to a significant decrease in tumor yield; and
- the tumor yield should be related to the dose of initiator while the efficacy and speed of tumor induction should be determined by the promoter.

Recently, more research efforts have been directed to development and evaluation of model systems that could be used for assessing the promotional activity of chemicals. While some of the methods are modelled on the original two-stage process of Berenblum, others measure end points which may correlate with the promotional capacity of the substance under test. Among this latter group are systems which measure aneuploidy induction in yeast cells (Parry et al., 1981), alterations affecting intercellular communication (Murray and Fitzgerald, 1979; Trosko et al., 1983; Williams, 1981), activation of viruses (Zur Hausen et al., 1979), induction or inhibition of cellular differentiation (Huberman and Callahan, 1979; Yamasaki et al., 1977) and induction of anchorage independent cell growth (Colburn et al., 1980). All of these systems are in the developmental stage and need to be evaluated before they can be recommended as routine screening procedures. There are also a number of *in vitro* and *in vivo* systems based on the two-stage model that are currently under investigation.

A number of studies have shown that *in vitro* transformation systems using $C3H/10T_{\frac{1}{2}}$ (Frazelle *et al.*, 1983; Mondal *et al.*, 1976; Sivak, 1982), BALB/c 3T3 (Sivak and Tu, 1980a) and Syrian hamster cells (Poiley *et al.*, 1979; Rivedal and Sanner, 1982) can be modified for such purposes and thus may be useful for evaluation of substances for promotional activity. In addition, *in vivo* systems have also been suggested for studying promotional events (Kroes, 1983; Weisburger and Williams, 1984). Model systems have been described for skin (Berenblum, 1974), stomach (Goerttler *et al.*, 1979), breast (Huggins *et al.*, 1961), liver (Farber and Sporn, 1976; Williams, 1982) and trachea (Topping and Nettesheim, 1980). Although these *in vivo* tests can provide quantitative information on promotional activity, a major disadvantage is their organ/tissue specificity.

V. Batteries of Short-Term Tests

Since a single test system does not provide an adequate perspective on the activity of a chemical, a battery of assays covering different end points and utilizing different metabolic capabilities is to be preferred for making an assessment of the mutagenicity or potential carcinogenicity of a chemical. However, from a consideration of our summary of the guidelines of international and national bodies as well as individuals, certain test systems can be identified as the most widely used. As there are a wide variety of applications for short-term tests, individual organizations may find it useful to tailor a battery of assays that will meet their specific needs for hazard identification.

The central principle in selecting a battery of tests is to choose various end points in different species ranging from bacteria to mammalian cells *in vivo*. This minimizes the possibility of failing to detect genotoxic activity while lending perspective to any single positive response. Assays utilizing prokaryotes provide an inexpensive, rapid testing procedure which yields preliminary indicators of genotoxic potential. For this as well as most other *in vitro* assays, a metabolic activation system such as a rat liver homogenate is required. Results from prokaryotic assays should be used in conjunction with results from other species and systems.

Assays utilizing mammalian cells may be more relevant than prokaryotes in predicting potential effects in man because of the presence of a nuclear chromosomal organization and different salvage and/or repair pathways. With these cells it is possible to measure a variety of genotoxic end points simultaneously and, in certain cases, effects in specific target cells in the whole animal.

In testing for genotoxic potential, it is advisable to include both a detection and risk assessment phase. The former phase is to determine if the chemical has genotoxic activity, and the latter is to determine the risk to man with respect to somatic and germinal mutations. In the detection phase, the battery should consist of at least four assays: a mutation assay in prokaryotic cells; a mutation assay in eukaryotic cells, preferably mammalian cells; an assay for chromosomal aberrations in mammalian cells; and an assay for DNA damage or its repair *in vivo* or *in vitro* such as UDS or SCE. In certain circumstances, such as low human exposure, not all these tests may be required. If the outcome from this testing indicates that the chemical is potentially genotoxic, additional testing is warranted with particular attention to those systems which provide information about heritable germ cell mutations or carcinogenesis.

It is recognized that *in vitro* transformation assays are difficult to perform, and there are limited studies on intra- and inter-laboratory reproducibility. Another point of concern is the limited metabolic capability of some of the cells used in the assay and the difficulty associated with incorporation of exogenous metabolic activation systems.

VI. Approaches to the Interpretation of Short-Term Test Results

There are a number of factors that should be taken into account in the overall evaluation and interpretation of results from short-term tests. A major consideration is what constitutes a positive or negative result in any assay. This will be determined by an evaluation of the specific protocol used and the criteria applied for defining and interpreting activity. Comparison of concurrent and historical controls as well as the influence of general nonspecific toxicity are also important elements in the interpretation of test results. As tests are developed, in order to carry out an adequate evaluation, it is essential that the test is an actual measure of a particular biochemical or biological phenomenon.

A review of the testing schemes indicates there is a general opinion that for reliable interpretation, results in multiple end points are needed (Section III). Once a suitable battery of short-term tests has been completed, careful analysis by experts is generally required in the interpretation of the data. This includes the application of sound statistical procedures in order to properly identify significant findings (Berstein *et al.*, 1982; Margolin *et al.*, 1981; Myers *et al.*, 1981; Snee and Irr, 1981; Stead *et al.*, 1981).

The first and most important point in the evaluation of short-term data is that despite the great similarities among all organisms at the molecular level, a positive response in any one test is not adequate for hazard evaluation and cannot, strictly speaking, be extrapolated to any other species or tissue. Nonetheless, such a positive effect in a single prokaryotic or eukaryotic mutagenicity assay suggests that the chemical may be genotoxic. Further research is required to resolve apparent conflict.

If all tests in a battery yield clear, positive results, then it is reasonable to regard that substance with a high level of concern for its mutagenic or carcinogenic potential in human beings. On the other hand, if a chemical is consistently negative in the battery, then it can be relegated to a lower level of concern as a human mutagen or carcinogen.

Since many agents appear to exert their carcinogenic effects through nongenotoxic mechanisms (Weisburger and Williams, 1980), the potential for carcinogenicity cannot be excluded on the basis of such negative findings. For such agents, other approaches to hazard identification are required (Grice *et al.*, 1984).

Unfortunately, the situation most commonly encountered in practice is that in which both positive and negative responses are observed among the various tests included in the battery. Furthermore, the particular pattern of responses may vary depending on the presence or absence of metabolic activation procedures used in conjunction with the tests. In these circumstances it may be difficult to draw a firm conclusion regarding level of concern, although the positive responses indicate some degree of mutagenic potential. For example, a chemical which is DNA-damaging, mutagenic and clastogenic should be regarded as a potential human carcinogen. Similarly, if an agent elicits only DNA damage and is mutagenic, this indicates that it is genotoxic and also, presumably, carcinogenic. Conversely, a weak positive result in one strain of *Salmonella* and clastogenic activity at high concentrations of the test substance *in vitro* may not generate the same level of concern.

In such cases, decisions as to further testing, use, or regulation of the material could be based largely on factors other than the actual test results themselves. Such factors include the exposure and use pattern of the particular chemical, its pharmacodynamics and details of its metabolic conversion patterns in humans, as well as the relative strength of the particular tests used in the battery for identification of hazard.

If the results in a battery of tests are equivocal and further evidence of carcinogenic potential other than a long-term bioassay is desirable, then a limited bioassay could be undertaken (Weisburger and Williams, 1978). This could involve the use of tests such as mouse skin initiation/ promotion, strain A mouse adenoma, enzyme markers in rat liver, neoplasm development in rat gastrointestinal tract or urinary bladder, and cell transformation. If the limited bioassay is positive, then it is likely that a chronic bioassay would also be positive. Conversely, if it is negative, a chronic study may still be required. In situations where dose-response data is necessary, the limited bioassay could be eliminated and a long-term bioassay undertaken.

Measures of potency. In principle, a numeric index of mutagenic potency may be calculated for any quantifiable genetic end point such as mutagenicity, DNA damage or clastogenicity. In cases where the dose-response relationship is linear, potency may be characterized in terms of the slope of the dose-response curve, with dose suitably standardized in terms such as molecular concentration (Horn *et al.*, 1983). It is important to recognize that in most systems, dose relates to cell exposure rather than the dose delivered to the target sites of interest. Possible approaches to this problem involve the use of equitoxic doses (Haynes and Eckardt, 1980) or molecular dosimetry to establish common doses for comparison (Lee, 1978). Another factor to be recognized is that there is no overall index of mutagenic potency for a substance tested in different systems. For example, in cell lines in which it is possible to measure simultaneously a variety of distinct genetic end points, considerable variation in potency of a given mutagen can be observed (Haynes *et al.*, 1982).

While such indices provide a convenient means of ranking different compounds according to their potency within a given assay, metabolic and cellular processes acting to modulate response *in vivo* make it difficult to extrapolate from *in vitro* test systems. For example, a highly potent *in vitro* mutagen which does not reach germinal cells would be ineffective *in vivo* on that tissue. Thus, in the absence of knowledge of the concentration of the test compound at the target site and the nature of the damage induced in different systems, predictions of mutagenic potency cannot be made with confidence.

Cancer development is a complex multi-step process involving many biological effects (Grice *et al.*, 1984). Thus, it is unlikely that any one effect observed in short-term tests would predict carcinogenic potency. Nevertheless, it has been suggested that bacterial mutagenicity may be quantitatively predictive of carcinogenicity (Meselson and Russell, 1977). While this may be true for some compounds, major discrepancies exist even within structurally similar classes of carcinogens. Indeed, for some assays such as the hepatocyte primary culture/DNA repair test, it has been pointed out that no quantitative correlation with carcinogenicity exists (Williams, 1977). Thus, potency in short-term tests should not be assumed to predict carcinogenic potency.

VII. Conclusions

During the last decade, short-term tests for chemical effects at the cellular and molecular level have undergone tremendous development. Well over 100 such tests for mutation, DNA repair synthesis, chromosomal aberrations, cell transformation or germ cell effects are now available for use. These tests may be used as predictors of genetic disease and carcinogenic potential, although the association between carcinogenic effects observed in long-term rodent bioassays and effects in short-term tests is somewhat inconsistent.

Our review of published guidelines on the use of short-term tests revealed a fair degree of agreement with respect to the use of certain tests. Most widely recommended were tests for mutation in prokaryotic organisms and cultured mammalian cells. In order to provide a fuller perspective on chemical activity, however, batteries of tests comprising different end points and metabolic capabilities are considered more suitable for hazard evaluation. In addition to the mutation of tests in prokaryotic and eukaryotic systems, assays for DNA damage and chromosomal aberrations in mammalian cells may be particularly useful for hazard identification.

Consistent positive results in a battery of short-term tests may be reasonably held to indicate a high degree of concern. While reassuring, negative results do not rule out the possibility of nongenotoxic mechanisms of carcinogenic action. Most difficult to interpret is the most common case in which both positive and negative results are encountered within the battery.

There is no doubt that short-term tests will continue to undergo vigorous development. New tests based on chromosomal rearrangements, DNA damage, cell transformation and promotional effects are on the horizon and may be expected to come into use in the near future. As these procedures become better understood, it is inevitable that they will play an increasingly important role in hazard assessment, possibly providing more definitive rather than supportive evidence of safety.

VIII. References

Adamkiewicz, J., Drosdziok, W., Eberhardt, W., Langenberg, U. and Rajewsky, M. (1982). High-affinity monoclonal antibodies specific for DNA components structurally modified by alkylating agents. In *Indicators of Genotoxic Exposure* (B.A. Bridges, B.E.

Butterworth and I.B. Weinstein, eds.), Banbury Reports 13, pp. 265-276, Cold Spring Harbor Laboratory, New York.

Ashby, J. (1983). The unique role of rodents in the detection of possible carcinogens and mutagens. *Mutat. Res.*, *115*, 77-213.

Berenblum, I. (1974). *Carcinogenesis as a Biological Problem* Elsevier/North Holland, New York.

Bermudez, E., Mirsalis, J.C. and Eales, H.C. (1983). Detection of DNA damage in primary cultures of rat hepatocytes following *in vivo* and *in vitro* exposure to genotoxic agents. *Environ. Mutagen., 4*, 667-679.

Berstein, L., Kaldor, J., McCann, J. and Pike, M.C. (1982). An empirical approach to the statistical analysis of mutagenesis data from the *Salmonella* test. *Mutat. Res., 97*, 267-281.

Bora, K.C. (1976). A hierarchical approach to mutagenicity testing and regulatory control of environmental chemicals. *Mutat. Res., 41*, 73-82.

Borek, C. (1983). Epithelial *in vitro* cell systems in carcinogenesis studies. *Ann. N.Y. Acad. Sci., 407*, 284-290.

Bridges, B.A. (1976). Use of a three-tier protocol for evaluation of long term toxic hazards particularly mutagenicity and carcinogenicity. In *Screening Tests in Chemical Carcinogenesis* (R. Montesano, H. Bartsch and L. Tomatis, eds.), pp. 549-568, International Agency for Research on Cancer, Lyon.

Bridges, B.A. (1973). Some general principles of mutagenicity screening and a possible framework for testing procedures. *Environ. Health Perspect., 6*, 221-227.

Bridges, B.A., Butterworth, B.E. and Weinstein, I.B. (eds.) (1982). *Indicators of Genotoxic Exposure* Banbury Report 13. Cold Spring Harbor Laboratory, New York.

Butterworth, B.E. (ed.) (1979). *Strategies for Short-term Testing for Mutagens/Carcinogens* CRC Press, West Palm Beach, Florida.

Butterworth, B.E., Earle, L.L., Strom, S.C., Jirtle, R.L. and Michalopoulos, G. (1983). Measurements of chemically induced DNA repair in human hepatocytes. *Proc. Am. Assoc. Cancer Res., 24*, 69.

Colburn, N.H., Koehler, B.A. and Nelson, K.J. (1980). A cell culture assay for tumor-promoter-dependent progression toward neoplastic phenotype: detection of tumor promoters and promotion inhibitors. *Teratogenesis, Carcinogenesis and Mutagenesis, 1*, 87-96.

Dean, B.J. (1976). A predictive testing scheme for carcinogenicity and mutagenicity of industrial chemicals. *Mutat. Res., 41*, 83-88.

Dean, B.J. (1983). The UKEMS sub-committee on guidelines for mutagenicity testing. *Mutat. Res., 113*, 527-529.

de la Iglesia, F.A., Lake, R.S. and Fitzgerald, J.E. (1980). Short-term tests for mutagenesis and carcinogenesis in drug toxicology: how to test and when to test is the question. *Drug Metab. Rev., 11*, 103-146.

Dixon, M. (1983). Report No. 16686. A yeast system for the detection of mutation recombination and aneuploidy. Lawrence Berkeley Laboratory.

Doolittle, D.J., Furlong, J., Earle, L.L. and Butterworth, B.E. (1983a). Measurement of chemically-induced DNA repair in human bronchial epithelium. *Pharmacologist, 25*, 174.

Doolittle, D.J., Sherrill, J.M. and Butterworth, B.E. (1983b). The influence of intestinal bacteria, sex of the animal, and position of the nitro group on the hepatic genotoxicity of nitrotoluene isomers *in vivo. Cancer Res., 43*, 2836-2842.

EEC (European Economic Community) (1980). Reports of the Scientific Committee for Food.

Emura, M., Richter-Reichhelm, H.B., Schneider, P., Scholch, C. and Mohr, U. (1982). Comparison of toxic and transforming effects of ten environment-related polycyclic hydrocarbons, including benzo(a)pyrene, on fetal hamster lung cell cultures. *J. Appl. Toxicol., 2*, 167-171.

EPA (Environmental Protection Agency) (1982). Pesticide registration; proposed data requirements. *Fed. Regis., 47*, 53192-53221.

Farber, E. and Sporn, M.B. (1976). Symposium: Early lesions and the development of epithelial cancer. *Cancer Res., 36*, 2476-2705.

Farmer, P.B., Bailey, E., Lamb, J.H. and Connors, T.A. (1980). Approach to quantitation of alkylated amino acids in hemoglobin by gas chromatography mass spectrometry. *Biomed. Mass Spectrom., 7*, 41-46.

FDA (Food and Drug Administration) (1982a). Chemical compounds in food-producing animals, availability of criteria for guidelines. *Fed. Regis., 47*, 4972-4977.

FDA (Food and Drug Administration) Bureau of Foods (1982b). Toxicological Principles for the Safety Assessment of Direct Food Additives and Color Additives Used in Food. U.S. Food and Drug Administration, Washington, D.C.

Flamm, W.G. (1974). A tier approach to mutagen testing. *Mutat. Res., 26*, 329-333.

Frazelle, J.H., Abernethy, D.J. and Boreiko, C.J. (1983). Factors influencing the promotion of transformation in chemically-initiated C3H/10T$\frac{1}{2}$ C18 mouse embryo fibroblasts. *Carcinogenesis, 4*, 709-715.

FSC (Food Safety Council) (1978). Proposed system for food safety assessment. *Food Cosmet. Toxicol., 16*, 1-109.

Goerttler, K., Loehrke, H., Schweizer, J. and Hesse, B. (1979). Systemic two-stage carcinogenesis in the epithelium of the forestomach of mice using 7,12-dimethylbenz(a)-anthracene as initiator and the phorbol ester 12-0-tetradecanoylphorbol-13-acetate as promoter. *Cancer Res., 39*, 1293-1297.

Grant, D. and Grasso, P. (1978). Suppression of Hela cell growth and increase in nuclear size by chemical carcinogens: a possible screening method. *Mutat. Res., 57*, 369-380.

Green, S. (1977). Present and future uses of mutagenicity tests for assessment of safety of food additives. *J. Environ. Pathol. Toxicol., 1*, 49.

Grice, H., Arnold, D., Clayson, D., Clarke, M., Emmerson, J., Fishbein, L., Hughes, D. and Krewski, D. (eds.) (1984). Interpretation and extrapolation of chemical and biological carcinogenicity data to establish human safety standards. In *Current Issues in Toxicology* Volume 2, Springer-Verlag, New York, 1984 (this volume).

Grimmer, G., Jacob, J., Schmoldt, A., Raab, G., Mohr, U. and Emura, M. (1983). Metabolism of benzo(a)anthracene in hamster lung cells in culture in comparison to rat liver microsomes. *Proc. Int. Symp. PAH No. 7*,, Ohio, in press.

Gupta, R.C., Reddy, M.V. and Randerath, K. (1983). Phosphorus-32-postlabelling analysis of non-radioactive aromatic carcinogen-DNA adducts. *Carcinogenesis*, *3*, 1081-1092.

Haynes, R.H. and Eckardt, F. (1980). Mathematical analysis of mutation induction kinetics. In *Chemical Mutagens, Principles and Methods for Their Detection* Volume 6, (F.J. de Serres and A. Hollander, eds.), pp. 271-308, Plenum Press, New York.

Haynes, R.H., Eckardt, F., Kunz, B.A. and Göggelmann, W. (1982). The importance of mutant yield data for the quantification of induced mutagenesis. In *Environmental Mutagens and Carcinogens* (T. Sugimura, S. Konda and H. Takebe, eds.), pp. 137-146, University of Tokyo Press, Tokyo.

Heidelberger, C., Freeman, A.E., Pienta, R.J., Sivak, A., Bertram, J.S., Casto, B.C., Dunkel, V.C., Francis, M.W., Kakunaga, T., Little, J.B. and Schechtman, L.M. (1983). Cell transformation by chemical agents - a review and analysis of the literature. A report of the U.S. Environmental Protection Agency Gene-Tox program. *Mutat. Res.*, *114*, 283-385.

Hollstein, M., McCann, J., Angelosanto, F.A. and Nichols, W.W. (1979). Short-term tests for carcinogens and mutagens. *Mutat. Res.*, *65*, 133-226.

Horn, L., Kaldor, J. and McCann, J. (1983). A comparison of alternative measures of mutagenic potency in the *Salmonella* (Ames) test. *Mutat. Res.*, *109*, 131-141.

Huberman, E. and Callahan, M.F. (1979). Induction of terminal differentiation in human promyelocytic leukemia cells by tumor-promoting agents. *Proc. Natl. Acad. Sci. U.S.A.*, *76*, 1293-1297.

Huggins, C., Grand, L.C. and Brillantes, F.P. (1961). Mammary cancer induced by a single feeding of polynuclear hydrocarbons, and its suppression. *Nature*, *189*, 204-207.

IARC (International Agency for Research on Cancer) (1980). *Monographs on the Evaluation of Carcinogenic Risk of Chemicals to Man*. Supplement 2: *Long-term and Short-term Screening Assays for Carcinogenesis: A Critical Appraisal*. IARC, Lyon.

ICPEMC (The International Commission for Protection Against Environmental Mutagens and Carcinogens) (1983). Committee 1 Final Report. Screening strategy for chemicals that are potential germ-cell mutagens in mammals. *Mutat. Res.*, *114*, 117-177.

Ishidate, M. (1983). Personal communication. National Institute of Hygienic Sciences, Tokyo.

Japan (1983). Toxicological guidelines for medical drugs in Japan (Draft guidelines). Toyko.

Kroes, R. (1983). Short-term tests in the framework of carcinogen risk assessment to man. *Ann. N.Y. Acad. Sci.*, *407*, 398-408.

Larsen, K.H., Brash, D., Cleaver, J.E., Hart, R.W., Maher, V.M., Painter, R.B. and Sega, G.A. (1982). DNA repair assays as a test for environmental mutagens. A report of the U.S. Environmental Protection Agency Gene-Tox program. *Mutat. Res.*, *98*, 287-318.

Lee, W. (1978). Dosimetry of chemical mutagens in eukaryote germ cells. In *Chemical Mutagens, Principles and Methods for Their Detection* Volume 5, (A. Hollander and F.J. de Serres, eds.), pp. 178-202, Plenum Press, New York.

Lutz, W.K. (1979). *In vivo* covalent binding of organic chemicals to DNA as a quantitative indicator in the process of chemical carcinogenesis. *Mutat. Res.*, *65*, 289-356.

Lucier, G.W. and Hook, G.E.R. (eds.) (1978). NIEHS Workshop: Higher plant systems as monitors of environmental mutagens. *Environ. Health Perspect.*, *27*, 1-206.

Margolin, B.H., Kaplan, N. and Zeiger, E. (1981). Statistical analysis of the Ames *Salmonella*/microsome test. *Proc. Natl. Acad. Sci. U.S.A.*, *78*, 3779-3783.

McQueen, C.A., Kreiser, D.A. and Williams, G.M. (1983). The hepatocyte primary culture DNA repair assay using mouse or hamster hepatocytes. *Environ. Mutagen.*, *5*, 1-8.

Meselson, M. and Russell, K. (1977). In *Origins of Human Cancer*, Book C (H.H. Hiatt, J.D. Watson and J.A. Winstein, eds.), p. 1473, Cold Spring Harbor Laboratory, New York.

Meyer, A.L. (1983). *In vitro* transformation assays for chemical carcinogens. *Mutat. Res.*, *115*, 323-338.

Mirsalis, J.C. and Butterworth, B.E. (1982). Induction of unscheduled DNA synthesis in rat hepatocytes following *in vivo* treatment with dinitrotoluene. *Carcinogenesis*, *3*, 241-245.

Mirsalis, J.C., Hamm, T.E., Jr., Sherrill, J.M. and Butterworth, B.E. (1982a). Role of gut flora in the genotoxicity of dinitrotoluene. *Nature*, *295*, 322-323.

Mirsalis, J.C., Tyson, C.K. and Butterworth, B.E. (1982b). Detection of genotoxic carcinogens in the *in vivo-in vitro* hepatocyte DNA repair assay. *Environ. Mutagen.*, *4*, 553-562.

Mishra, N., Dunkel, V.C. and Mehlman, M. (eds.) (1980). *Advances in Modern Environmental Toxicology* Volume 1, Senate Press, New Jersey.

Mondal, S., Brankow, D.W. and Heidelberger, C. (1976). Two-stage chemical oncogenesis in cultures of C3H/10T$\frac{1}{2}$ cells. *Cancer Res.*, *36*, 2254-2260.

Murray, A.W. and Fitzgerald, D.J. (1979). Tumor promoters inhibit metabolic cooperation in cocultures of epidermal and 3T3 cells. *Biochem. Biophys. Res. Commun.*, *91*, 395-401.

Myers, L.E., Sexton, N.H., Southerland, L.I., Wolff, T.J. (1981). Regression analysis of Ames test data. *Environ. Mutagen.*, *3*, 575-586.

NCI (National Cancer Institute) (1981). Cameron, T. Personal communication.

Netherlands (Health Council of the Netherlands) (1982). Summary of the report on the mutagenicity of chemical substances. pp. 1-14.

Newbold, R.F., Overell, R.W. and Connell, J.R. (1983). Induction of immortality is an early event in malignant transformation of mammalian cells by carcinogens. *Nature*, *299*, 633-635.

NTP (National Toxicology Program) (1982). NTP Technical Bulletin. Issue No. 6, p. 2.

OECD (Organization for Economic Cooperation and Development (1983). OECD data interpretation guides for initial hazard assessment. Paris, France.

OSHA (Occupational Safety and Health Administration) (1980). Identification, classification and regulation of potential occupational carcinogens. *Fed. Regis.*, *45*, 5001-5296.

Pai, S.B., Steele, V.E. and Netteshiem, P. (1982). Identification of early carcinogen-induced changes in nutritional and substrate requirements in cultured tracheal epithelial cells. *Carcinogenesis*, *3*, 1201-1206.

Painter, R.B. (1977). Rapid test to detect agents that damage human DNA. *Nature*, *265*, 650-651.

Parry, J.M., Parry, E.M. and Barrett, J.C. (1981). Tumour promoters induce mitotic aneuploidy in yeast. *Nature*, *294*, 263-265.

Petzold, G.L. and Swenberg, J.A. (1978). Detection of DNA damage induced *in vivo* following exposure of rats to carcinogens. *Cancer Res.*, *38*, 1589-1594.

Poiley, J.A., Raineri, R. and Pienta, R.J. (1979). Two-stage malignant transformation in hamster embryo cells. *Br. J. Cancer*, *39*, 8-14.

Popescu, N.C., Amsbaugh, S.C. and DiPaolo, J.A. (1980). Enhancement of N-methyl-N'-nitro-N-nitrosoguanidine transformation of Syrian hamster cells by a phorbol diester is independent of sister chromatid exchanges and chromosome aberrations. *Proc. Natl. Acad. Sci. U.S.A.*, *77*, 7282-7286.

Purchase, I.F.H. (1982). An appraisal of predictive tests for carcinogenicity. *Mutat. Res.*, *99*, 53-71.

Ray, V.A. (1979). Application of microbial and mammalian cells to the assessment of mutagenicity. *Pharmacol. Rev.*, *30*, 537-546.

Rivedal, E. and Sanner, T. (1982). Promotional effect of different phorbol esters on morphological transformation of hamster embryo cells. *Cancer Lett.*, *17*, 1-8.

Roberts, J.J. (1976). Possible diagnostic value of caffeine on an inhibitor of post replication DNA repair of chemically modified DNA: enhancement of toxicity, chromosome damage and effects on newly synthesized DNA. In *Screening Tests in Chemical Carcinogenesis* (R. Montesano, H. Bartsch and L. Tomatis, eds.), p. 605, International Agency for Research on Cancer, Lyon.

San, R.H.C. and Stich, H.F. (eds.) (1980). *Short-Term Tests for Chemical Carcinogens* Springer-Verlag, New York.

Sega, G.A. (1982). DNA repair in spermatocytes and spermatids of the mouse. In *Indicators of Genotoxic Exposure* Banbury Reports 13. (B.A. Bridges, B.E. Butterworth and I.B. Weinstein, eds.), pp. 503-514, Cold Spring Harbor Laboratory, New York.

Shimada T., Furukawa, K., Kreiser, D.M., Cawein, A. and Williams, G.M. (1983). Induction of transformation by six classes of chemical carcinogens in adult rat liver epithelial cells. *Cancer Res.*, *43*, 5087-5092.

Silinskas, K.C., Kateley, S.A., Tower, J.E., Maher, V.M. and McCormick, J.J. (1981). Induction of anchorage-independent growth in human fibroblasts by propane sultone. *Cancer Res.*, *41*, 1620-1627.

196   Short-Term Tests for Mutagenicity and Carcinogenicity

Sivak, A. (1982). An evaluation of assay procedures for detection of tumor promoters. *Mutat. Res., 98*, 377-387.

Sivak, A. and Tu, A.S. (1980a). Factors influencing neoplastic transformation by chemical carcinogens in BALB/c 3T3 cells. In *The Predictive Value of In Vitro Short-term Screening Test in Carcinogenicity Evaluation* (G.M. Williams, R. Kroes, H.W. Waaijers and K.W. van de Poll, eds.), pp. 171-190, Elsevier/North Holland, Amsterdam.

Sivak, A. and Tu, A.S. (1980b). Cell culture tumor promotion experiment with saccharin, phorbol myristate acetate and several common food materials. *Cancer Lett., 10*, 27-32.

Snee, R.D. and Irr, J.D. (1981). Design of a statistical method for analysis of mutagenesis of the hypoxanthine-guanine phosphoribosyl transferase locus of cultured Chinese hamster ovary cells. *Mutat. Res., 85*, 77-93.

Sobels, F.H. (1980). Evaluating the mutagenic potential of chemicals. The minimal battery and extrapolation problems. *Arch. Toxicol., 46*, 21-30.

State of California (1982). Carcinogen identification policy: a statement of science as a basis for policy. State of California Health and Welfare Agency. pp. 1-57.

Stead, A.G., Hasselbald, V., Creason, J.P. and Claxton, L. (1981). Modeling the Ames test. *Mutat. Res., 85*, 13-27.

Stoltz, D.R., Poirer, L.A., Irving, C.C., Stich, H.F., Weisburger, J.H. and Grice, H.C. (1974). Evaluation of short-term tests for carcinogenicity. *Toxicol. Appl. Pharmacol., 29*, 157-180.

Stoltz, D.R., Stavric, B., Krewski, D., Klaassen, R., Bendal, R. and Junkins, B. (1982). Mutagenicity screening of foods. 1. Results with beverages. *Environ. Mutagen., 4*, 477-492.

Swenberg, J.A. and Bedell, M.A. (1982). Cell-specific DNA alkylation and repair: application of new fluorometric techniques to detect adducts. In *Indicators of Genotoxic Exposure* Banbury Report 13, (B.A. Bridges, B.E. Butterworth and I.B. Weinstein, eds.), pp. 205-220, Cold Spring Harbor Laboratory, New York.

Topping, D.C. and Nettesheim, P. (1980). Promotion-like enhancement of tracheal carcinogenesis in rats by 12-O-tetradecanoylphorbol-13-acetate. *Cancer Res., 40*, 4352-4355

Trosko, J.E., Jone, C. and Chang, C. (1983). The role of tumor promoters on phenotypic alterations affecting intercellular communication and tumorigenesis. *Ann. N.Y. Acad. Sci., 407*, 316-327.

United Kingdom (1981). *Guidelines for the Testing of Chemicals for Mutagenicity. Report on Health and Social Subjects*. pp. 1-95, Department of Health and Social Security, London.

Waters, M.D., Simmon, V.F., Mitchell, A.D., Jorgenson, T.A. and Valencia, R. (1980). An overview of short-term tests for the mutagenic and carcinogenic potential of pesticides. *J. Environ. Sci. Health*, Part B. Pesticides, Food contaminants and agricultural wastes. *B15(6)*, 867-906.

Weisburger, J.H. and Williams, G.M. (1978). Decision point approach to carcinogen testing. In *Structural Correlates of Carcinogenesis and Mutagenesis* (I.M. Asher and C. Zervos, eds.), pp. 45-52, Office of Science, Food and Drug Administration, Maryland.

Weisburger, J.H. and Williams, G.M. (1980). Chemical carcinogens. In *Toxicology: The Basic Science of Poisons 2nd Edition*, (J. Doull, C.D. Klaassen and M.O. Amdur, eds.), pp. 84-138, Macmillan, New York.

Weisburger, J.H. and Williams, G.M. (1981). Carcinogen testing: current problems and new approaches. *Science, 214*, 401-407.

Weisburger, J.H. and Williams, G.M. (1984). Bioassay of carcinogens: *in vitro* and *in vivo* tests. In *Chemical Carcinogens* (C.E. Searle, ed.), American Chemical Society, Washington, D.C.

Williams, G.M. (1977). Detection of chemical carcinogens by unscheduled DNA synthesis in rat liver primary cell cultures. *Cancer Res., 37*, 1845-1851.

Williams, G.M. (1980). Batteries of short-term tests for carcinogen screening. In *The Predictive Value of In-Vitro Short-term Screening Tests in Carcinogenicity Evaluation* (G.M. Williams, R. Kroes, H.W. Waaijers and K.W. van de Poll, eds.), pp. 337-346, Elsevier/North Holland, Amsterdam.

Williams, G.M. (1981). Liver carcinogenesis: the role for some chemicals of an epigenetic mechanism of liver tumor promotion involving modification of the cell membrane. *Food Cosmet. Toxicol., 19*, 577-583.

Williams, G.M. (1982). Phenotypic properties of pre-neoplastic rat liver lesions and applications to detection of carcinogens and tumor promoters. *Toxicol. Pathol., 10*, 3-10.

Williams, G.M. (1983). Genotoxic and epigenetic carcinogens: their identification and significance. *Ann. N.Y.Acad. Sci., 407*, 328-333.

Williams, G.M. and Weisburger, J.H. (1981). Systematic carcinogen testing through the decision point approach. *Ann. Rev. Pharmacol. Toxicol., 21*, 393-416.

Working, P.K. and Butterworth, B.E. (1982). An *in vivo-in vitro* assay to detect chemically-induced DNA repair in spermatogenic cells. *J. Cell Biol., 95*, 171a.

Yamasaki, H., Fibach, E., Nudel, U., Weinstein, I.B., Refkind, R.A. and Marks, P.A. (1977). Tumor promoters inhibit spontaneous and induced differentiation of murine erythroleukemia cells in culture. *Proc. Natl. Acad. Sci. U.S.A., 74*, 3451-3455.

Zur Hausen, H., Bornkamm, G.W., Schmidt, R. and Hecker, E. (1979). Tumor initiators and promoters in the induction of Epstein-Barr virus. *Proc. Natl. Acad. Sci. U.S.A., 76*, 782-785.